Medical Anthropology and African American Health

Medical Anthropology and African American Health

Eric J. Bailey

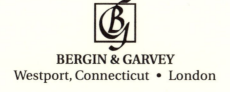

BERGIN & GARVEY
Westport, Connecticut • London

Library of Congress Cataloging-in-Publication Data

Bailey, Eric J., 1958–
    Medical anthropology and African American health / Eric J. Bailey.
      p. cm.
    Includes bibliographical references and index.
    ISBN 0–89789–592–4 (alk. paper)
    1. Afro-Americans—Health and hygiene—Social aspects.   2. Afro-
Americans—Medical care—Social aspects.   3. Medical anthropology.
    4. Health and race—Social aspects.   I. Title.
    [DNLM: 1. Anthropology, Cultural—methods—United States.
    2. Blacks—United States.   3. Ethnic Groups—United States.
    4. Health Behavior—ethnology—United States.   5. Health Services
Needs and Demand—United States.   6. Health Services Research—
methods—United States.   WA 300 B154m   1999]
    RA448.5.N4B424   2000
    362.1′089′96073—dc21
    DNLM/DLC   99–21244

British Library Cataloguing in Publication Data is available.

Library of Congress Catalog Card Number: 99–21244
ISBN: 0–89789–592–4

First published in 2000

Bergin & Garvey, 88 Post Road West, Westport, CT 06881
An imprint of Greenwood Publishing Group, Inc.
www.greenwood.com

Printed in the United States of America

The paper used in this book complies with the
Permanent Paper Standard issued by the National
Information Standards Organization (Z39.48–1984).

10 9 8 7 6 5 4 3 2 1

Excerpts from Eric Bailey's "Medical Anthropologist as Health Department Consultant" *Practicing Anthropology* (Winter 1994, Volume 16, Number 4) are reprinted with permission from The Society for Applied Anthropology.

To the memory of my grandparents
Roger William Bailey, Sr. and Ollie Glanton Bailey
And
John Lee Ballew and Lula Chenault Ballew

Contents

Preface

Medical Anthropology and African American Health is a teaching text and resource guide for students, health care professionals, health care researchers, and the general public that explains the relationship of culture to African American health care issues. The major emphasis of this book is a *cultural relativistic* approach to health care assessment, intervention and implementation programs designed especially for African Americans. "Cultural relativistic" refers to the concept of understanding and evaluating an individual and/or a group from his/her or the group's perspective.

Specifically, Chapter 1 discusses the field of medical anthropology and describes how the approach of medical anthropology is particularly appropriate for today's African American health care issues. Chapter 2 shows how the health beliefs and treatment actions of other identified U.S. ethnic minority populations are similar to African Americans' health beliefs and treatment actions.

Chapter 3 discusses African American health from a comprehensive, holistic sociocultural perspective. It explains African American culture within a cultural historical context. Chapter 3 highlights also the current and often neglected sociodemographic factors associated with the African American population and it describes how psychosocial factors such as religiosity/spirituality influence health. Finally, it shows how cultural historical health incidents have affected African Americans' perception of the U.S. health care system.

Chapter 4 highlights the major causes of death among African Americans and how culture is related to each disease. Chapter 5 describes African Americans' alternative medical practices from the perspective of their history, their health belief system, and their treatment patterns. Chapter 6 discusses the basic strategies for conducting applied medical anthropology studies. Qualitative ethnographic strategies used in clinical, public health, and community settings are highlighted. In addition, ethical issues are discussed in the context of being an African American health care researcher who studies African Americans.

Chapters 7 through 14 highlights the author's applied medical anthropological studies conducted in clinical, public health, and community-based settings. These studies were conducted from 1982 to 1995. Each study shows how the author developed his particular style of conducting applied medical anthropology regardless of the setting or number of participants in the study.

Chapter 15 highlights successful programs that have used a cultural relativistic approach to health care intervention for specific African American groups such as the African American elderly, African American women, African American men, African American adolescent females, and African American adolescent males. In addition, the author suggests a number of cultural health empowerment strategies for health care professionals, health care researchers, public health administrators, and patients.

Each chapter begins with Critical Thinking Questions and ends with Post-Evaluation Questions.

Acknowledgments

I want to express my sincere appreciation to all the students in my classes during the past fifteen years. Their insight and comments have encouraged me to develop a new approach to the field of medical anthropology and African American health. I also thank Sally Crisp, EdD. for her collegial evaluation of this book manuscript. Her expertise and comments were very much appreciated. In addition, I want to thank Jane Garry, Nina Duprey, Bonnie Kaplan, and all the staff members at Greenwood Publishing.

To conduct fieldwork in communities, clinics, and public health settings requires cooperation with local agencies and key informants. I want to express my thanks for all those who have assisted me in each fieldwork project. Individuals such as Helen Kinard, Shannon Jones, Anne Helton, Joe Rubio, Gershom Gamor, Lynnette Rodriquez, Laura Williams, and Debbie Thomas were invaluable key informants. Cooperative agencies such as the Cincinnati Health Department, Bethesda Hospital, Henry Ford Hospital, Houston Health Department, the March of Dimes Texas Gulf Coast Chapter, the Regenstrief Health Clinic, St. Joseph Hispanic Health Services, SisterLove Inc., Miami University (Ohio), Central State University (Ohio), Wayne State University, Emory University School of Public Health, the University of Arkansas for Medical Sciences, Indiana State Health Department, and IUPUI's Faculty Development Office also provided their support.

Finally, I wish to thank all my family members and friends (past and present) for their personal opinions about health care and the African American community. In particular, I wish to thank my outstanding parents, Roger and Jean Bailey and my brothers, Dwight, Ronnie, Billie, and Michael for their lifelong encouragement, support, and inspiration. I am grateful to Gloria, Ebony, and Darrien for their continual support, patience, and passion for learning.

Part I

Medical Anthropology, Culture and Ethnic Populations Health Issues

Your journey into the field of medical anthropology begins with a broad discussion of this academic discipline and its approach to the health care field. An overview of the history, the early theoretical orientations from various scholars, and the major subdisciplines of medical anthropology are all presented. Most importantly, the reader discovers how medical anthropology can be used to solve today's critical medical and health care issues in the United States and globally. Culture is the crosscutting theme that establishes the field of medical anthropology as separate from a majority of the medical and health care disciplines. The concept of culture and its relationship to health is the major emphasis throughout the entire book.

Chapter 1

Medical Anthropology and Health Care

CRITICAL THINKING QUESTIONS

1. Describe the unique approach of medical anthropology to health care.

2. What are the types of health research projects of interest to medical anthropologists?

3. Describe the relationship of culture with health care issues.

INTRODUCTION

What Is Medical Anthropology?

Medical anthropology is often poorly understood by those who are not a part of the discipline. When working with other health care professionals, medical anthropologists are commonly asked to explain what their field is, what they do, and how they can assist clinicians and public health officials in appropriating better health care for their patients/clients. Many assume that medical anthropologists are on excavations like archaeologists or that we are very similar to biologists.

Medical anthropology focuses on disease, illness, medical problems, theories of illness, and health care systems in different cultural and ethnic groups from a

biopsychosociocultural perspective (Figure 1.1). In other words, medical anthropologists investigate health care from a holistic perspective. We attempt to

Figure 1.1
Biopsychosociocultural Perspective

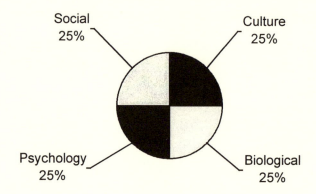

to take a broader approach than other disciplines in order to ensure that all the
possible factors are sufficiently investigated.

The biopsychosociocultural perspective means exactly what the term states.
That is, one must recognize the biological, psychological, social, and cultural
factors that are connected with each individual as they relate to health or illness.
Therefore, the biopsychosociocultural model provides a blueprint for research, a
framework for teaching, and a design for action in the real world of health care.

Medical anthropology is actually a subspecialty field of anthropology. Anthropology refers to the study of human behavior; medical anthropology, then,
focuses upon the biology, psychology, sociology, cultural, and medical aspects
of human behavior. Those who specialize in this subspecialty are referred to as
medical anthropologists or applied medical anthropologists. The major difference between the two terms is that the applied medical anthropologist attempts
to operationalize the theory, concept, and approach into tangible outcomes,
whereas the medical anthropologist simply describes and analyzes various
medical aspects of human behavior.

Medical Anthropology Research Issues and African American Health

The field of medical anthropology is such a broad-based subspecialty that it
offers the medical anthropologist a vast array of research areas to investigate.
Research topics of interest range from investigating ethnic and/or cultural

groups' definitions of health and disease, to determining how to improve a doctor's relationship with an ever more diverse patient population.

The field of medical anthropology can be used to examine the following critical African American health care issues.

1. Breast Cancer
- Investigate the high rates of breast cancer among African American women;
- Examine the social and cultural barriers in seeking breast cancer information and participating in screening programs; and
- Develop culturally competent breast cancer intervention programs for African American women.

2. Adolescent Smoking Pattern
- Investigate the reasons African American adolescents have a lower prevalence rate of cigarette smoking when compared to European American adolescents;
- Examine the social and cultural factors that influence the lower prevalence rate of cigarette smoking among African American adolescents; and
- Develop culturally competent smoking cessation programs for African American adolescents and adults.

3. Diabetes
- Investigate the reasons African Americans have high prevalence rates of diabetes;
- Examine the social and cultural barriers in seeking diabetes information and adhering to a diabetic regimen; and
- Develop culturally competent diabetes intervention programs for African Americans.

4. Stroke
- Investigate the reasons African Americans have high prevalence rates of strokes;
- Examine the social and cultural factors to stroke prevention programs; and
- Develop culturally competent stroke prevention programs for African Americans.

5. Asthma
- Investigate the reasons African Americans have high prevalence rates of asthma;
- Examine the social and cultural factors that influence their high prevalence rates; and
- Develop culturally competent asthma prevention programs for African Americans.

Photo 1.1
Eric Bailey Teaching Medical Anthropology at Indiana University, Bloomington –
Summer 1989

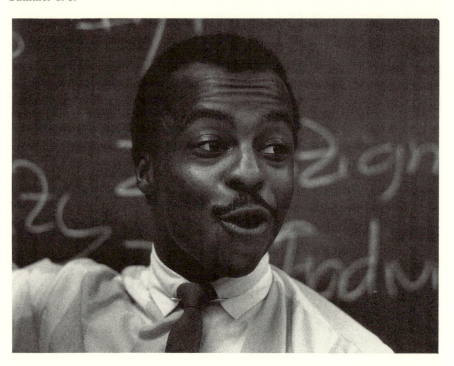

6.   Prostate Cancer
- Investigate the reasons African American men have high prevalence rates of prostate cancer;
- Examine the social and cultural barriers in seeking prostate cancer information; and
- Develop culturally competent prostate cancer intervention programs for African American men. (U.S. Department of Health and Human Services 1997).

Additional questions that are of major interest to medical anthropologists are as follows:

1.   How are older people cared for in different cultural and ethnic groups?
2.   How do cultural and ethnic groups treat mentally ill persons?
3.   How are people "recruited" or "trained" as practitioners, and how are the "roles" learned, completed, and changed?

4. Why are alternative medical practices used in varying degrees by a majority of the population?
5. What is the relationship between pattern of life and pattern of disease among certain segments of the population? and
6. How can a local, regional, or national health care agency develop culturally appropriate and culturally competent health care programs?

These questions highlight a few of the research questions that most medical anthropologists try to address in their research and applied endeavors.

The History of Medical Anthropology

The field of medical anthropology developed from a long-standing interest of anthropologists in health care systems in non-Western societies. Historically, medical anthropology can be traced to three distinct sources:

1. The traditional ethnographic interest in "indigenous" or "native" medicine among non-Western peoples;
2. The culture and personality movement within anthropology in the 1930s and 1940s and the beginning of collaborative studies by psychiatrists and anthropologists; and
3. The growth of the international public health movement following World War II and the increased interest in the application of modern health care systems in developing countries.

Theoretical Approaches of Medical Anthropology

This section reviews chronologically the major theorists who contributed to the theoretical orientation in medical anthropology. Since the 1920s, three major empirical generalizations have emerged as underlying themes from all the theories:

1. Disease in some form is a universal fact of life; it occurs in all known times, places, and societies.
2. All known human groups develop methods and allocate roles, congruent with their resources and structures, for coping with, or responding to, disease.
3. All known human groups develop some set of beliefs, cognitions, perceptions, consistent with their cultural matrices, for defining or recognizing disease. (Wellin 1977:48)

In other words, the early medical anthropology theorists recognized not only that diseases occur in all societies but that it was also important to acknowledge the belief and treatment practices among all known human groups. The theorists who were often recognized for this type of perspective to medical care consisted of individuals such as W.H.R. Rivers, Forrest Clements, Erwin Ackerknecht, Benjamin Paul, and ecological theorists.

W.H.R. Rivers

William Hallam Rivers attempted to relate systematic native medicine to other aspects of culture and social organization. In such works as *Medicine, Magic, and Religion* (1924) and *Psychology and Ethnology* (1926), Rivers formulated two themes: first, primitive medical practices follow from and make sense in terms of, underlying medical beliefs, and second, native and primitive medical practices are best conceived not as quaint folklorisms but as integral parts of culture. Based on this general proposition, he developed a model that defines three types of worldviews and associated belief systems with three corresponding modes of behavior. In this model, Rivers emphasizes the importance of the magical and religious worldviews of native cultures.

Although most medical anthropologists view Rivers' model as static and nonapplicable, Rivers recognized that the fundamental elements of native medicine constitute a social institution and he understood that the interrelationships between native medical practice and belief constitute integral parts of a culture.

Forrest Clements

In his monograph, "Primitive Concepts of Disease" (1932), Clements classifies disease causation concepts among native peoples into five categories:

1. sorcery,
2. breach of taboo,
3. intrusion by a disease object,
4. intrusion by a spirit, and
5. spirit loss.

Clements documents these categories of disease causation by illustrating their worldwide distribution. From these categories, Clements formulates his model.

His model contends that diffusion and/or historic-geographic events produce given profiles of distribution for each disease concept that determine the time sequences and courses of spread for each. Thus, disease causation concepts are culturally derived at a specific time period and do not undergo adaptive changes (Clements 1932).

Despite the limits of Clement's model, he illustrates that societies everywhere develop some set of cognitions for defining disease. Clement's approach inspired Ackerknecht to elaborate on the importance of a culture's concept of disease causation.

Erwin Ackerknecht

Although Ackerknecht's research was primarily from libraries and museum documents rather than from ethnographic fieldwork, his works had a powerful shaping influence on the framework of medical anthropology. Ackerknecht's five generalizations are as follows:

1. The responses of a given sociocultural and medical system to the introduction of new elements are to be explained not solely by the nature of the system nor alone by the nature and mode of introduction of a new element but by the complex interaction of both.
2. There are not one native medicine but many native medicines, perhaps as many as there are native cultures.
3. The parts of the medical pattern, like those of the entire culture, are functionally interrelated, although the degree of functional integration of elements at both levels varies from one society to another.
4. Native medicine is best understood largely in terms of cultural belief and definition, that is, without consideration of biologic, epidemiologic, and environmental factors.
5. The varied manifestations of native medicine are based on magic medicine (Wellin 1977:52).

Benjamin Paul

Benjamin Paul's theoretical orientation represents an important departure from the approach of Rivers, Clements, and Ackerknecht. The major difference concerns Paul's "applied" strategy, which addressed the dynamic nature of different cultural medical systems. Paul's model is based on two fundamental propositions:

1. The responses of a given sociocultural and medical system to the introduction of new elements are to be explained not solely by the nature of the system nor alone by the nature and mode of introduction of a new element but by the complex interaction of both.
2. Reciprocal or feedback processes occur. That is, the introduction of new health-related elements can be expected to affect the host sociocultural and medical systems; in turn, the latter also affects (shapes or reinterprets) the new elements. (Wellin 1977:53)

The importance of Paul's system-model is that it includes the medical systems of modern or complex communities for analyses as well as those of a traditional group. Paul's system-model is a dynamic model that addresses the nature and consequences of change. In other words, social factors such as economics and education as well as cultural factors such as beliefs and disease causation and treatment practices influence the type of care people receive from their medical and health care system and, in turn, help to shape new methods of health care intervention.

Ecological Approach

Although medical anthropology benefited greatly from Paul's system-model in the 1950s, the ecological approach has contributed most to the discipline. From the early 1960s to the present, ecological orientation is a dominant theme in the field of medical anthropology. The ecological orientation views health and disease from a biological and cultural perspective with respect to the culture's environment.

Studies such as Livingstone's classic study (1958) of the sickle-cell trait in West Africa, Wiesenfeld (1967) of Malaysia's agricultural system affecting the rates of the sickle-cell trait and malaria, and McCracken's study (1971) of the worldwide distribution of lactose intolerance have enlightened health care researchers and professionals about the impact of environment on one's health status. Additionally, McElroy and Townsend's (1996) *Medical Anthropology in Ecological Perspective*, Brown's (1998) *Understanding and Applying Medical Anthropology*, and Baer, Singer, and Susser's (1997) *Medical Anthropology and the World System* provide current examples of the ecological approach to medical anthropology. In general, the ecological orientation of medical anthropology emphasizes the interrelationship between environmental factors and health.

Subdisciplines of Medical Anthropology

The four major subdisciplines of medical anthropology are:

1. Ecology and epidemiology
2. Medical aspects of the health care system
3. Medicine and culture change and
4. Ethnomedicine

These four major subdisciplines of medical anthropology provide the medical anthropologist with the tools and skills to examine health behavioral science issues from a holistic and comprehensive perspective.

Ecology and epidemiology investigate primarily the distribution, dynamics, and frequencies of disease occurrences in relationship to the environmental setting. In this subdiscipline, the medical anthropologist asks the following questions regarding a health care issue: (1) What environmental or social factors increase the prevalence of a certain disease pattern within a particular ethnic group? (2) Are there any cultural health patterns practiced within a particular cultural and/or ethnic group that influence or contribute to the disease pattern? These questions are essential areas to investigate primarily because the medical anthropologist can uncover subtle or overt cultural health patterns that are connected to the distribution and frequencies of certain diseases.

The second major subdiscipline of medical anthropology is referred to as the medical aspects of the health care system. This subdiscipline focuses upon illness or disease within a society and determines whether or not it is an indicator of the health care system performance. In other words, high rates of disease and/or illnesses within a given social health care system are an indication that the local and national health care system does not perform well. Some medical anthropologists would say that the high rates of preventable diseases such as heart disease, cancer, cerebrovascular diseases, HIV/AIDS, tuberculosis, unintentional injuries, and infant mortality are an example of the ineffectiveness of the U.S. health care system. In contrast, some medical anthropologists would say that the continual increase in life expectancy for U.S. citizens (e.g., 74 years for males, 78 for females) is an indication that the U.S. health care system is providing the U.S. population with a longer life.

The third major subdiscipline, medicine and culture change, refers to the process whereby populations modify and adapt their traditional health care practices to the health care practices and treatment therapies of the majority population. Studies show that populations migrating from rural to urban or from non-Western to Westernized society tend to add new health care practices while still retaining their traditional health care practices (Landy 1977). Those populations that have a good balance between the new health care practices and the old health care practices tend to maintain good healthy outcomes. Yet those populations that adopt primarily the urban or Westernized health care practices tend to experience serious health care consequences.

Finally, ethnomedicine, the fourth major subdiscipline of medical anthropology, highlights the major difference of medical anthropology compared to other behavioral science disciplines. Ethnomedicine is the study of how members of different cultural and/or ethnic groups "think" about disease/illness and how they "organize" themselves toward treatment. The medical anthropologist is primarily concerned with two major issues: (1) the individual's and/or group's perception of the illness and (2) the individual's and/or group's pattern of treatment practices. Investigating these two issues leads the medical anthropologist to discover the cultural factors related to the individual's or group's health-seeking process.

Subdisciplines of Anthropology

1. Physical anthropology
2. Archaeology
3. Linguistics and
4. Cultural Anthropology

Each subdiscipline is unique in its approach and perspective.

Physical anthropology is the subdiscipline of anthropology that focuses upon the biological, physical, and genetic characteristics of human populations. Those who specialize in physical anthropology study past and present human populations' physical and genetic characteristics. Oftentimes, physical anthropologists' goals are (1) to compare early and present-day populations' physical characteristics; (2) to analyze disease patterns from different time periods and different populations in order to find the pattern and distribution of certain disease; and (3) to develop ergonomically designed products for specific populations based on their anthropometric measurements. Additional areas of concentration within physical anthropology are human osteology, human evolution, medical genetics, and human physical variation.

Archaeology is another major subdiscipline of anthropology. Archaeology attempts to reconstruct and analyze material remains of human populations. Whether of past or present–day populations, archaeologists reconstruct a picture of the daily lifestyle and behavioral patterns of human populations by examining the objects people have manufactured.

The third major subdiscipline of anthropology is linguistics, the study of language patterns of cultural and ethnic groups. Within the subdiscipline of linguistic anthropology are three subspecialties: descriptive linguistics, historical linguistics, and sociolinguistics. These three subspecialties provide a comprehensive analysis of language. For instance, descriptive linguistics investigates how language is constructed. It examines the basic structure of each type of language system. It focuses upon speech sounds, grammar, syntax, and the semantics of each language system. Historical linguistics, on the other hand, investigates the origins and changing patterns of language systems. Finally, sociolinguistics examines the impact of social and cultural factors upon language patterns.

The fourth and final subdiscipline of anthropology is sociocultural anthropology. Sociocultural anthropology examines all the elements of society that influence human behavior, such as economics, education, kinship, politics, technology, social norms and values, and health care. Sociocultural anthropology is closely linked to medical anthropology primarily because of its holistic approach to understanding human behavior.

Culture and Health: The Field of Anthropology

Anthropology is a discipline unlike any other discipline in academe. Anthropology examines human populations from a holistic and comprehensive perspective. Anthropology is a study of human populations not only from a biological, physical, or genetic approach but also from a sociocultural perspective. That is, anthropologists study the everyday behavioral patterns of human cultures and how various socioeconomic or cultural factors influence our behavioral patterns. Thus, anthropology is quite distinct from other disciplines.

The four major, distinctive qualities of anthropology that set it apart from other disciplines are:

1. it's holistic;
2. it requires fieldwork;
3. it's comparative; and
4. it examines culture.

Let's see how anthropology is different from other disciplines.

The father of american anthropology, Franz Boas (1940), and many of his students such as Zora Neale Hurston (1942) and Margaret Mead (1928), was one of the early anthropologists who always emphasized the holistic and comparative approach. Holism is an approach well established in anthropology since its foundation. The holistic approach attempts to analyze as many factors as possible to account for human behavior. By using this approach, the anthropologist can determine which factors (biological, psychological, or cultural) influence human behavior patterns more often than others do. It also provides the anthropologist with awareness of how all these factors interrelate to affect human behavior. In other words, the holistic approach gives the anthropologist a broader perspective on how populations exist and function on a daily basis.

The second major, distinctive quality is that anthropology requires fieldwork. An anthropologist must conduct ethnographic fieldwork outside a controlled environment. That is the community is usually our field of investigation, not a laboratory or controlled office setting where experimental testing is conducted. The anthropologist, therefore, is at the mercy of his or her fieldwork setting. Learning how to adapt and to conduct ethnographic research in the field is a skill that all anthropologists need.

The third major distinctive quality is comparative. Anthropology is naturally comparative in its approach simply because of our analyses of different cultural and ethnic groups. Anthropology is the only discipline that constantly examines other cultural and ethnic groups in an attempt to understand behavioral patterns. By doing this, eventually, anthropologists are able to develop some significant universal themes and patterns that are common among all human populations.

The fourth and final major, distinctive quality of anthropology is the concept of culture. The word "culture" is used quite often to describe a wide array of human behavioral patterns. In this book, culture is defined as a system of shared beliefs, values, customs, and behaviors that are transmitted from generation to generation through learning.

The major attributes of culture are:

1. it's a learned process;
2. it's transmitted by symbols;
3. it adds meaning to reality;
4. it's differently shared;
5. it's integrated; and most importantly,
6. it's adaptive (Figure 1.2)

Culture relates directly to health care in the following ways. For instance, all of us learn a particular pattern of taking care of ourselves, we learn a certain health belief system, we learn when to take a health care action, and we learn when to seek care from others.

Medical anthropologists recognize the connection between culture and symbols. The culture of health care is transmitted by a wide array of symbols. In the health care field, symbols may refer to one's diagnosis (e.g., HBP = high blood pressure), symbols may refer to the type of health care organization (e.g., CDC = Centers for Disease Control and Prevention or DHHS = Department of Health and Human Services), or symbols may be verbal (e.g., the nonverbal signals between doctor and patient that convey a good rapport and relationship versus a poor rapport and mistrust).

Figure 1.2
Culture Attributes

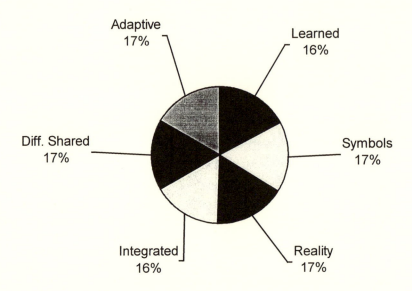

Medical anthropologists recognize also the interrelationship between culture and its meaning to the health care field. In the health field, individuals go through years of learning and training to achieve their particular specialty in medicine or nursing (e.g., medical doctor, clinical nurse, licensed nurse, physician's assistant). Once the individual completes his or her training, he or she is certified with a degree and recognized by society to practice his or her specialized skill in health care.

Medical anthropologists recognize also that the culture of health care is differently shared. All of us experience different perceptions of the local and national health care system. Some experiences are good whereas other experiences are poor. These perceptions vary widely from one person to another.

Medical anthropologists recognize also that the culture of health care is integrated. That is, our local and national health care system is closely intertwined with other elements of society such as economics, politics, social issues, and cultural perceptions of quality health care. Thus, health care is integrated into the total sociocultural fabric of our society.

Finally, medical anthropologists recognize that the culture of health care is adaptive. Our health care system continues to change every year in an attempt to meet the demands and needs of our ever-growing and diverse population.

CONCLUSION

The field of medical anthropology is a discipline that incorporates the perspective of a wide range of approaches. It is a discipline that takes these various approaches to health care from anthropologists, sociologists, epidemiologists, medical doctors, nurses, public health administrators, biologists, and the general public and attempts to bring all these elements together in an effort to better understand the health care issues of the past, present, and future. This is the very reason that medical anthropology uses the biopsychosociocultural approach to health care.

The biopsychosociocultural approach is a holistic, flexible, ever-changing, and adaptable model to the health care field. This model provides a blueprint for research, a framework for teaching, and a design for action in the real world of health care (Engel 1977).

In this book, I emphasize the cultural component of the biopsychosociocultural model due to the fact that there has been little attention to culture and its relationship to health and the difficulty of defining culture as it relates to a particular population. *Culture* is the driving force or essential component to this model.

POST-EVALUATION QUESTIONS

1. How can medical anthropology be used in your project or setting?

2. How can culture influence health care decisions?

3. How can each subfield of medical anthropology contribute to the health care field?

REFERENCES

Ackerknecht, Erwin. 1971. *Medicine and Ethnology: Selected Essays.* Baltimore: Johns Hopkins University Press.

Adair, J., and K. Deuschle. 1970. *The People's Health.* New York: Appleton-Century Crofts.

Alland, Alexander. 1977. "Medical Anthropology and the Study of Biological and Cultural Adaptation." In *Culture, Disease and Healing*, David Landy, ed. Pp. 41–47. New York: Macmillan.

Anderson, Robert. 1996. *Magic, Science, and Health: The Aims and Achievements of Medical Anthropology.* Fort Worth, TX: Harcourt Brace College Publishers.

Baer, Hans, Merrill Singer and Ida Susser. 1997. *Medical Anthropology and the World System: A Critical Perspective.* Westport, CT: Bergin & Garvey.

Boas, Franz. 1940. *Race, Language, and Culture.* New York: Macmillan.

Brown, Peter. 1998. *Understanding and Applying Medical Anthropology.* Mountain View, CA: Mayfield.

Clements, Forrest. 1932. "Primitive Concepts of Disease." *American Archeology and Ethnology* 32:185–252.

Engel, George. 1977. "The Need for a New Medical Model: A Challenge for
    Biomedicine." *Science* 196:129–136.
Hurston, Zora Neale. 1942. *Dust Tracks on a Road*. Philadelphia: Lippin-
    cott.
Kaplan, D., and R. Manner. 1972. *Culture Theory*. Englewood Cliffs, NJ:
    Prentice-Hall.
Kleinman, A., L. Eisenberg, and B. Good. 1978. "Culture, Illness and Care:
    Clinical Lessons from Anthropologic and Cross-Cultural Research."
    Annals of Internal Medicine 88:251–258.
Kluckhohn, C. 1945. "The Personal Document in Anthropological Science." In
    Use of Personal Documents in History, Anthropology and Sociology, L.
    Gottschalk, C. Kluckhohn, and R. Anglell, eds. U.S. of America, Social
    Science Research Council. New York: Committee on Appraisal of Re-
    search.
————. 1962. *Culture and Behavior*. New York: Free Press of Glencoe.
Landy, David. 1977a. *Culture, Disease and Healing*. New York: Macmillan.
————. 1977b. "Role Adaptation: Traditional Curers under the Impact of
    Western Medicine." In *Culture, Disease and Healing*. David Landy, ed.
    Pp. 468–480. New York: Macmillan.
Leininger, Madeleine. 1970. *Nursing and Anthropology. Two Worlds to Blend*.
    New York: John Wiley and Sons.
————. 1978. *Transcultural Nursing: Concepts, Theories and Practices*.
    New York: John Wiley and Sons.
Lieban, R. 1977. "The Field of Medical Anthropology." In *Culture, Disease and
    Healing*, David Landy. ed. Pp. 12–31. New York: Macmillan.
Livingstone, Frank. 1958. "Anthropological Implications of Sickle-Cell Gene
    Distribution in West African." *American Anthropologist* 60:533–562.
Malinowski, Brownislaw. 1922. "Ethnology and Study of Society." *Economica*
    2:208–219.
McCracken, Robert. 1971. "Lactase Deficiency: An Example of Dietary
    Evolution." *Current Anthropology* 12:479–517.
McElroy, Ann, and Patricia Townsend. 1996. *Medical Anthropology in
    Ecological Perspective*. Third ed. Boulder, CO: Westview Press.
Mead, Margaret. 1928. *Coming of Age in Samoa*. New York: William Morrow.
Paul, Benjamin. 1955. *Health, Culture, and Community: Case Studies of Public
    Reactions to Health Programs*. New York: Russell Sage Foundation.
————. 1963. "Anthropological Perspectives on Medicine and Public Health."
    Annals of the American Academy of Political and Social Science
    346:34–43.
Rivers, Williams Hallam. 1924. *Medicine, Magic and Religion*. London:
    Kegan Paul, Trench, Trubner.
————. 1926. *Psychology and Ethnology*. London: Harcourt Brace Jovanovich.
U.S. Department of Health and Human Services. 1997. *Health, United States
    1996-7 and Injury Chartbook*. National Center for Health Statistics.
    Washington, DC: U.S. Government Printing Office. DHHS Publication
    No. 97–1232.
Wellin, E. 1977. "Theoretical Orientations in Medical Anthropology: Change
    and Continuity over the Past Century." In *Health and the Human*

Condition: Perspectives on Medical Anthropology, Michael Logan and
Edward Hunt, eds. Pp. 23–39. North Scituate, MA, Duxbury Press.
Wiesenfeld, S.L. 1967. "Sickle-Cell Trait in Human Biological and Cultural
Evolution." *Science* 157:1134–1140.

WEB SITES OF SIGNIFICANCE

American Anthropology Association

http://www.ameranthassn.org

Anthropology and Medicine

http://www.carfax.co.uk/anm-ad.htm

Medical Anthropology Quarterly

http://www.ameranthassn.org/smapubs.htm

Social Science and Medicine

http://www.elsevier.com/inca/publications/store/3/1/5

Society for Applied Anthropology

http://www.telepath.com/sfaa

Society for Medical Anthropology

http://www.people.memphis.edu~sma

Chapter 2

Ethnic Populations in the United States: Health Beliefs and Treatment Actions

CRITICAL THINKING QUESTIONS

1. To what degree do health beliefs affect ethnic groups' utilization of health services?

2. Why do ethnic groups vary in their health beliefs and treatment actions?

3. Do ethnic groups share common health beliefs and treatment actions to similar illnesses?

INTRODUCTION

Anthropologically, ethnic groups are defined as "those who share a sense of cultural and historical uniqueness, and to act as a member of an ethnic group is to express feelings or call attention to that uniqueness" (Mindel and Habenstein 1981). There is a degree of conformity and commonality of those who share this social and cultural heritage. It is expressed in a variety of ways, such as physical appearance, language, kinship organization, speech patterns, food traditions, long-standing rituals, religious belief systems, and in particular, health beliefs and treatment actions.

Oftentimes, the definitions of ethnic groups and minority groups have been misconstrued and misunderstood. Unlike the term "ethnic groups," the concept of minority groups conveys another set of sociocultural issues. For instance, "minority" refers to a power or dominance relationship. Those groups that have unequal access to power or health care, that are considered in terms of assumed inferior traits or characteristics are minority groups. To be a member of a minority group, then, is to share a status relationship, and to act as a minority group member is to express power (Mindel and Habenstein 1981).

It is therefore imperative that we understand the difference between these two terms—ethnicity and minority—and how these two terms affect individuals who are a part of these groups. Additionally, if one is a part of a particular ethnic group and unfortunately labeled by society as part of a minority group, being a part of both groups has a direct impact on one's health beliefs, treatment patterns, and health-seeking process.

HEALTH-SEEKING PROCESS

Health-seeking process is a concept that describes the events that take place when a person is sick. This behavioral pattern includes steps taken by an individual who perceives a need for help as he or she attempts to solve a health problem (Chrisman 1977). The following steps are conceptually differentiated as elements in the health-seeking process.

1. Healthy,
2. Symptom definition,
3. Illness-related shifts in role behavior,
4. Lay consultation and referral,
5. Treatment actions, and
6. Adherence (Bailey 1991; Chrisman 1977).

The first element, healthy, consists of the pattern that an individual takes to maintain his or her health. Preventive health practices vary widely with each individual and group and are directly related to one's sociocultural situation. Preventive health practices are also related to one's folk health belief system. What individuals think about maintaining good health and how they go about it are directly related to their folk/traditional preventive health care pattern.

According to the health-seeking process, an individual's symptom definition develops when the degree of discomfort becomes noticeable and acknowledgeable by his or her cultural group. If the illness receives a cultural stamp, then a health care action follows (Chrisman 1977). Cultural stamp refers to an agreed-upon understanding and acceptance of a situation by those who share similar beliefs and values.

Illness-related shifts in role behavior are the third stage of the health-seeking process. This stage refers to the change or adaptation in the behavior of the sick or ill person. Whether the individual continues his or her daily activities or not is highly dependent on the ethnic/cultural group's definition of an ill/sick person.

The fourth stage lay consultation and referral, is the individual's familial, friend, or social network in seeking health care information. The lay consultation and referral network outside the household is likely to derive initially from friends and/or relatives as opposed to health care professionals.

The major reasons individuals may utilize extensively their informal lay consultation and referral network for health care problems are that

1. the reciprocal give-and-take relationship between the individual and family, friends, neighbors, or acquaintances can act as a buffer between the individual and the stressful situation;
2. these sources can alleviate the stress by helping the person instrumentally or by helping the person psychologically better cope with the situation; and
3. there is the opportunity for everyone to be involved in the healing process (Bailey 1991).

The fifth stage, treatment actions, is likely to vary for the individual according to class, region of the United States, and degree of assimilation to mainstream society. Most individuals have the option of selecting from a variety of sources, such as

1. formal health professionals;
2. licensed health practitioners;
3. alternative or native health practitioners;
4. lay consultation; and
5. self.

Studies have shown that ethnic minority populations tend to consult an alternative or native health practitioner primarily because of

1. their attempt to cope with health problems within the context of their resources and sociocultural/ethnic environment;
2. their belief that alternative health practitioners have some control over the forces that cause anomalies in a person's life, whereas Westernized physicians cannot help certain cause of illness and misfortune; and
3. lower monetary expense associated with such treatments (Cockerham 1986, Hill 1976; Bailey 1991).

The final step of the health-seeking process, adherence, refers to the degree to which the sick person acts upon the treatment advice. The adherence of ethnic groups to traditional remedies as well as the difficulty some patients have in understanding the biomedical presentation of physicians affect not only the quality of care but also the adherence to prescribed treatment regimens.

This overview of the health-seeking process illustrates how sociocultural and ethnic factors may influence an individual's health care action. This framework of ethnic health beliefs and treatment actions provides a basis for understanding the ethnic and sociocultural bond an individual may develop toward his or her health beliefs and treatment actions. The health-seeking process model should be considered only a framework for understanding ethnic health beliefs and treatment actions, not an absolute, structured model for understanding the multi-faceted approach connected to health seeking.

The following sections of Chapter 2 examine the health beliefs and treatment actions of the three major racial and ethnic populations in the United States: Hispanic/Latino Americans, Asian and Pacific Islanders, and American Indians and Alaskan Natives. The major purpose in examining the health beliefs and treatment actions of these three racial and ethnic populations in the United States is to show how similar their ethnic health belief system is to African Americans' health belief system and also to show how cultural historical factors influence each ethnic group's health belief system. In the following chapters, African Americans' health belief system is thoroughly examined.

HISPANIC/LATINO AMERICANS

Hispanic/Latino Americans' Culture and Sociodemographics

The Hispanic/Latino American population is the second largest ethnic minority group (U.S. Department of Commerce 1993). The term "Hispanic" is an umbrella term used to conveniently describe a large and diverse population. Hispanics constitute 10.0% of the population, with 19.4 million living in the United States. A person with a Hispanic background is one who conditions and events surrounding and influencing his or her life, including education, language, experiences, and health beliefs are associated with Spanish civilization (*Latin American Wave* 1997). We must realize that each Hispanic group is distinct and unique, with its own history. Each group has its own relation to this country, and each tends to be concentrated in different geographic areas of the United States (Vazquez and Ramirez-Krodel 1989:2).

The United States' Hispanic/Latino population (Figure 2.1) is divided into five main subgroups: Mexican Americans (62.3%), Puerto Ricans (12.7%), Cuban Americans (5.3%), Central and South Americans (11.5%), and people of other Hispanic origin (8.1%).

Eighty-seven percent of Hispanics live in urban areas. Cuban Americans most often live in Florida, while Mexican Americans live primarily in the western states. Most Puerto Ricans reside in Puerto Rico and New York (U.S. Department of Commerce 1993; Vazquez and Ramirez-Krodel 1989).

Two important and related sociodemographic facts about the Hispanic population include its youthfulness and its birthrate. The median age of the Hispanic population is 25.5, compared to 32.9 for the total population. Also, the birthrate for Hispanics was 23.3 per 1,000 women in 1989, while the birthrate for the total U.S. population was 15.5 births per 1,000 women (U.S. Department of Health and Human Services 1997).

Hispanic/Latino American Health Beliefs and Practices

Due to the lack of cultural health data about the five main subgroups of the Hispanic/Latino population, this section can examine comprehensively only three of the five main Hispanic racial and ethnic groups' traditional health beliefs and practices: Mexican Americans, Puerto Ricans, and Cuban Americans. Although there are similarities in the ways in which Mexican Americans, Puerto Ricans, and Cuban Americans perceive health and illness and in the use of folk healers and remedies, documented research studies have shown some distinct differences. Therefore, this section highlights the significant health issues related to the traditional health beliefs and practices of Mexican Americans, Puerto Ricans, and Cuban Americans.

Figure 2.1
United States' Hispanic Population - Five Main Subgroups

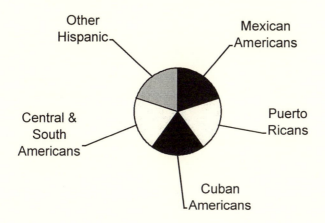

History: Mexican Americans

Depending on socioeconomic status, age, and the area in which one lives, a member of this large minority group may refer to himself or herself as either Mexican American, Spanish American, Latin American, Latin, or Latino (Simmen 1972). The term "Chicano" is used as an "identifying umbrella that identifies all Americans of Mexican descent"—a term accepted more on the West Coast and Midwest, but not as much in Texas and its neighboring states. (Simmen 1972).

Mexican Americans have been in the United States for a long time, moving from Mexico and later intermarrying with Indians and Spanish people in the southwestern parts of what is now the United States. Most of the descendants of these early settlers now live in Arizona, California, Colorado, New Mexico, and

Texas (Spector 1985). A large number of Mexican Americans also live in Illinois, Indiana, Kansas, Michigan, Missouri, Nebraska, New York, Ohio, Utah, Washington, and Wisconsin. Most Mexican Americans arrived in the latter states as migrant farmworkers. While located there as temporary farmworkers, they found permanent jobs and stayed (Simmen 1972). Contrary to the popular views that Mexican Americans live in rural areas, most live in urban areas. In fact, today, California and Texas still constitute the largest population centers for Mexican Americans (U.S. Department of Commerce 1993).

History: Traditional Health Beliefs

According to the Hippocratic theory, the body humors (blood, phlegm, black bile, and yellow bile) vary in both temperature and moistness. In this system, health is conceived as a state of balance among the four humors that manifests itself in a somewhat wet, warm body. Illness, on the other hand, is believed to result from a humoral imbalance that causes the body to become excessively dry, cold, hot, wet, or a combination of these states. Food, herbs, and other medications, which are classified as wet or dry, hot or cold, are used therapeutically to restore the body to its supposed natural balance. Thus, according to the system, a "cold" disease, such as arthritis, is cured by administering "hot" foods or medications (Harwood 1971; Spector 1985; Spicer 1979). However, there is no general agreement as to what is a hot disease or food and what is a cold disease or food. In addition, the classification varies from person to person, and what is hot to one person may be cold to another (Saunders 1954).

The hot-cold system stems from the Hippocratic humoral theories of disease, which were carried to the Western Hemisphere by the Spanish and Portuguese in the sixteenth and seventeenth centuries (Harwood 1971). Medical schools established in Mexico and Peru in this period taught the system, and its tenets were also embodied in household medical references and Aztec beliefs, which were used throughout Spanish America by priests and others who provided European medical care to the indigenous populations (Lucero 1975). Through these channels of influence, the humoral theory became an integral part of Mexican American folk medical practice, where it persists today (Harwood 1971; Spector 1985).

The hot-cold syndrome in Latin America has been reported for Mexico, for Mexican American communities, for the Guatemalan Highlands, for coastal Colombia, for the Colombian Highlands, and for coastal Peru and coastal Chile (Beals 1946; Foster 1953; Clark 1959; McFeeley 1949; Saunders 1954; Rubel 1960; Simmons 1972; Currier 1966). For example, cold foods include most fresh vegetables, the ancient Indian staples (maize, beans, and squash), most tropical fruits (including citrus fruits), dairy products, and low-prestige meats such as goat, fish, and chicken. Hot foods include most (but not all) chili peppers, most temperate-zone fruits, goat's milk, cereal grains, high-prestige meats such as beef, waterfowl, most oils, hard liquor, and aromatic beverages. A given food stuff is often both hot and cold, depending on whether and how it is cooked. Foods that can be either hot or cold are beans, rice, wheat, pork, and peaches (Currier 1966).

The qualities of hot and cold are related to aspects of life other than those of nutrition and disease. In these other contexts the symbolic meanings of warmth and cold are most clearly revealed: cold is associated with threatening aspects of existence, while warmth is associated with reassurance (Madsen 1955; Rubel 1960; Currier 1966; Ingham 1970; Spicer 1979).

In sum, the traditional framework of knowledge about health and disease of Mexican Americans is integrated by a conceptualization of the individual as a sum of balanced parts and qualities (Rubel 1960). A healthy individual is one whose entire being is in balance. This concept relates to the set of contrasting qualities, hot and cold, wet and dry. Conceptually, individuals and parts of their body are conceived as having specific place and function; a change in the manner in which any of these parts relates to the whole is presumed to cause illness.

Health-Seeking Process

Mexican Americans: Symptom Definition

According to the health-care seeking model, an individual's symptom definition develops when the degree of discomfort becomes noticeable and acknowledgeable by his or her ethnic and/or cultural group. If illness receives a cultural stamp, then a health care action follows (Chrisman 1977). Mexican American folk medicine classifies disease mainly according to cause rather than symptoms. The primary classification of disease distinguishes three major categories:

1. natural and supernatural forces;
2. imbalances of hot and cold; and
3. emotions as a cause of disease (Chesney, Thompson, and Guevara 1980; Klein 1978; Abril 1977; Kiev 1968).

Natural and supernatural forces cause diseases either by an individual's violating the balance of the natural world controlled by God or by a bewitchment sent by human adversaries utilizing evil, satanic forces. A natural illness is corrected by restoring the particular balance that was disrupted. Bewitchment is cured by countermagic or by removing the immediate source of harm (Madsen 1964).

For example, exposure to the forces of nature, such as moonlight, eclipses, cold, heat, air, wind, sun, and water, is believed to cause illness (Abril 1977; Kay 1979). "Mal aire" is a folk belief in which "bad air" affects children and adults, causing pain and cramps (Clark 1959). "Bad air" may enter the body of a child or an adult, producing aches in the particular area where it lodges. Thus, it is a health belief to protect oneself from cold winds and night air (Madsen 1964).

In terms of the supernatural forces, some people believe that some ailments are caused by magical powers such as the "evil eye." If someone with "strong vision" admires someone else's child without actually touching him or her, the child may fall ill—the evil power is transmitted through the gaze of that person. Symptoms of this illness include insomnia, aches and pains, excessive crying, fever, severe headache, and restlessness. All individuals are regarded as susceptible to the virulence of "evil eye" (mal ojo) but women and children are more receptive than men are (Rubel 1960).

Imbalances of hot-cold are the second major cause of disease among Mexican Americans. The state of health is seen as demanding a balance between the hot and cold and maintaining a strong defense against outside forces. Some diseases are hot, and some are cold. In addition, foods and herbs are classified into hot and cold treatments (Abril 1977; Rubel 1960; Kay 1979). Sickness that enhances the cold within the body requires a hot treatment to restore the balance, and vice versa. To avoid a hot sickness, the person must not become cold; therefore the individual must not walk barefoot on cold tiles for fear of catching tonsillitis (Ripley 1986). Moreover, people are given chili, a hot food, or chicken soup for a cold disease such as pneumonia or a common cold.

Finally, emotions as a cause of disease are the third major category. An example of an emotionally based illness is called *susto*. Susto (fright) is usually the result of a traumatic experience that may be anything from witnessing an accident or death to a simple scare at night (Spector 1985; Rubel 1977). It afflicts many people—males and females, rich and poor, rural dwellers and urbanities. It involves "soul loss": the soul is able to leave the body and wander freely. This can occur while a person is dreaming or when a person experiences a particularly traumatic event. Often, the susto syndrome will appear in which an individual is unable to meet the expectations of his or her own society for a social role in which he or she has been socialized (Rubel 1977). The symptoms of the disease are as follows:

1. The person is restless while sleeping.
2. When awake, the person is listless, anorexic, and disinterested in personal appearance, which includes both clothing and personal hygiene.
3. The person experiences a loss of strength, is depressed, and becomes introverted (Spector 1985).

Mexican American Treatment Actions

The types and sources of treatment actions among Mexican Americans, Puerto Ricans, and Cuban Americans are likely to vary according to gender, age, class, region of the United States, and degree of assimilation to mainstream society. In the United States, most ethnic groups have the option of selecting from the variety of sources as listed earlier.

In addition to the variety of home remedies or patent medicines used among Mexican Americans, a variety of alternative health practitioners serve the Mexican American community: (1) sobador, (2) curandero, (3) yerbero, (4) espiritisa, and (5) santero. Each alternative health practitioner uses different treatment actions.

For example, the sobador (massager) is usually a woman who gives therapies rather than medicines (Kay 1979). She is needed in cases of indigestion, infection (empacho), or counseling. The curandero, on the other hand, is a full-time or part-time specialist who heals by virtue of a "gift from God," typically revealed and confirmed in dreams and often involving a close association with the spirit of a renowned predecessor. Curanderos, who may be male or female (curandera), often see themselves as having unusual qualities, thereby obtaining a high status within the community (Edgerton 1970). Curanderos also rub, massage, and otherwise manipulate the body (e.g., "lifting" the fontanelle back into place). Still other curanderos have occult powers, including the ability to bewitch as well as to cure (Foster and Anderson 1978).

The yerbero (herbalist), espiritisa (practitioner of Espiritism, a religious cult concerned with communication with spirits and the purification of the soul through moral behavior), and santero (practitioner of Santeria, a religious cult concerned with teaching people how to control or placate the supernatural) are the other major alternative health practitioners serving the Mexican American community (Randall-David 1989). Each of these alternative health practitioners plays an important role in the Mexican American community.

Finally, many Mexican American alternative treatment patterns do not require alternative healers or home remedies. For many illnesses, Mexican Americans frequently seek the intervention of saints, the Virgin, or Christ, lighting candles and praying at their alters. Often, vows or solemn promises are made to "miraculous" images of Christ or the Virgin. All in all, Christ and the Virgin are only advocates who intercede for their human clients; God, in the final analysis, decides on the outcome (Foster and Anderson 1978:76).

Sociodemographics: Puerto Ricans and Cuban Americans

Of the five main Hispanic American racial and ethnic groups, Puerto Ricans consist of approximately 12.5% and Cuban Americans approximately 4.9% of the population. Puerto Ricans residing on the mainland (United States) live mostly on the East Coast, with the greatest number living in New York City and metropolitan New Jersey. Cuban Americans, on the other hand, are clustered predominantly in New York and southern Florida (U.S. Department of Commerce 1993; Stern 1993).

In addition, Puerto Ricans and Cuban Americans constituted one of the most recent immigration waves to the United States. Many are Catholic, but some belong to Protestant sects (Spector 1985).

Puerto Rican and Cuban American Traditional Health Beliefs

There are similarities in the ways in which Puerto Ricans, Cuban Americans, and Mexican Americans perceive health and illness and in the use of folk healers and remedies. There are also slight differences that need to be addressed.

For example, when the Hippocratic theory was incorporated into Latin American folk practice, the wet-dry dichotomy became insignificant as a basis for diagnostic and therapeutic decisions, and the hot cold (*caliente-frio*) dimensions came to dominate the system (Harwood 1971). In the Puerto Rican and

Cuban cultural variant of the system, diseases are grouped into hot and cold classes, while medications and foods are categorized as hot, cold, or an intermediate category, "cool" (*fresco*) (Harwood 1971; Steward 1956; Padilla 1956). Cold-classified illnesses are treated with hot medication and foods, while hot illnesses are treated with cool substances (Harwood 1971).

While there is general agreement about the assignment of foods and medicines to the hot-cold classifications, the system allows for variation. In general, a person may categorize a food or medicine differently from the norm if it individually produces physical symptoms that are typically classified as hot or cold (Spector 1985; Harwood 1971). For instance, a person may note that pineapple causes diarrhea or some other hot reaction (e.g., hives) and therefore considers it hot (*caliente*), even though it is not generally so considered. Pork is a food that is particularly subject to variant categorization.

In sum, the traditional framework of knowledge about health and disease among Puerto Ricans and Cuban Americans is very similar to Mexican Americans' traditional health and disease framework. The very fact that new items are still being incorporated into the hot-cold classification and an intermediate category (cool) attests to the vitality of the Puerto Ricans' and Cuban Americans' traditional health beliefs and practices.

Health-Seeking Process

Puerto Ricans and Cuban Americans: Symptom Definition

The categories of disease causation among Puerto Ricans and Cuban Americans are quite similar to Mexican Americans' folk diseases. Common colds, however, are seen as quite serious by many Puerto Ricans, since they are viewed as the start of a possible chain of illnesses, brought on by repeated chills and failure to effect a cure (Harwood 1971). Thus, an untreated or chronic cold is believed to lead to chronic shortness of breath or wheezing (fatiga), which, in turn, may develop into bronchitis or even tuberculosis.

Other examples in which the proper hot-cold balance in the body is of importance include (1) a baby should not be fed a formula (hot), as it may cause rashes; whole milk (cold) is acceptable; (2) a person who has been working (hot) must not go into the coffee fields (cold), or he or she can contract a respiratory illness; and (3) a hot person must not drink cold water, as it could cause colic (Spector 1985).

Puerto Ricans and Cuban Americans: Treatment Actions

Puerto Ricans and Cuban Americans practice many of the same treatment actions as Mexican Americans. Nonetheless, one particular alternative health practitioner, the *santero*, has been documented frequently to serve the Puerto Rican community. The *santero* is an important person: he respects the individual and does not gossip about either the person or his or her problems. Anyone can "pour his or her heart out" with no worry of being labeled or judged. The *san-*

tero is able to tell a person what the problem is, prescribe the proper treatment, and tell the person what to do, how to do it, and when to do it (Spector 1985).

Conclusion

This section highlights the significant health beliefs and practices among Mexican Americans, Puerto Ricans, and Cuban Americans. Although there is little documented research on all the five main subgroups of Hispanics, the literature on alternative medicine, especially among Mexican Americans, Puerto Ricans, and Cuban Americans, suggests that the choice of conventional care and/or alternative medicine depends on the symptom, that families often use both alternative and conventional medicine, that they are more likely to seek medical help for anxiety than for depression, and that knowledge of alternative medicine is best acquired by asking about specific folk diseases (Ailinger 1985; Chesney et al. 1980; Mayers 1989; Rivera 1988; Trotter 1991; Rosa 1988).

This brief review of the health beliefs and practices in the Mexican American, Puerto Rican, and Cuban American cultures reflects a broader understanding of the factors that influence their health action (Bailey 1987; Warren 1992; Saunders 1991; U.S. DHHS 1985). Moreover, the cultural-historical analysis of Mexican American, Puerto Rican, and Cuban American traditional health beliefs and practices provides a special insight regarding the ethnic and sociocultural bond an individual may develop toward his or her health beliefs and practices.

As former U.S. Department of Health and Human Services, director, Louis Sullivan (1992) stated at the National Workshop on Hispanic/Latino Health, there are five major areas that we need to focus on if we are going to improve the health and health status of the Hispanic/Latino community:

1. We need to enhance access to health care;
2. We need to improve the data collection on the Hispanic/Latino population;
3. It is imperative that we increase Hispanic representation in the sciences and health professions;
4. We need to focus greater attention and resources on health promotions and disease prevention; and
5. We need to emphasize calls for comprehensive and relevant research for the Hispanic/Latino populations.

ASIAN AND PACIFIC ISLANDER AMERICANS

Asian and Pacific Islander American Culture and Sociodemographics

This section highlights the significant health issues associated with Asian and Pacific Islander Americans. Due to the lack of cultural health data about each Asian American and Pacific Islander group, this section summarizes the major points of interest.

Asian Americans are defined as the federally designated minority populations whose origins are the Far East, Asia, and Southeast and Southwest Asia. Individuals of Asian descent who are U.S. citizens or permanent residents residing in the United States are considered Asian Americans. According to the 1990 Census designations, Asian Americans include, but are not limited to, those who self-classify themselves to be Asian Indians, Cambodians, Chinese, Filipino, Hmong, Japanese, Korean, Laotian, Thai, Vietnamese, and "other Asian" (Min 1995).

Pacific Islander Americans are defined as individuals who are descendants of the original residents of the Pacific Islands under the jurisdiction of the U.S. government. According to the 1990 Census designations, these individuals include, but are not limited to, Chamorro, Hawaiians (Kanaka Maoli), Melanesians, Micronesians, Polynesians, Samoans, and "other" Pacific Islanders (Chamorros are the people indigenous to Guam, and Kanaka Maoli are the indigenous Hawaiians).

The number of Asian and Pacific Islander Americans in the United States grew 120 percent between 1970 and 1980. As of 1980, Asian and Pacific Islander Americans numbered 3.7 million and constituted 1.6% of the population. Asian and Pacific Islander Americans come from more than twenty different countries. The three most common countries of origin are China, the Phillippines, and Japan (U.S. Department of Health and Human Services 1985).

Additional sociodemographics of importance are the mean age and mean educational. The median age of the Asian and Pacific Islander American is 28.7 years and the median educational level is similar to that of the general population. Three out of four have completed high school, and approximately one out of three holds a college degree (U.S. Department of Health and Human Services 1985).

History: Asian Americans

During the past few decades, the growth of the Asian American population has primarily resulted from changes in U.S. immigration law enacted in 1965 and to the flood of refugees from Vietnam, Laos, and Cambodia following the fall of South Vietnam in 1975. Asians in very small numbers entered the United States as early as the late eighteenth century. During the late nineteenth and early twentieth centuries, fair numbers of Chinese, Japanese, Korean, and then Filipino farm laborers were brought to California and Hawaii, so a very small Asian American minority was visible (Barringer, Gardner, and Levin 1993; Min 1995).

Historically, in 1860 the only Asian American group of any significance in the United States was the Chinese. Their numbers grew rapidly until 1880, after which the Chinese Exclusion Act cut off most immigration from China. Following the 1965 changes in the immigration laws, growth skyrocketed to over 1.6 million Chinese Americans. Presently, Chinese Americans have been the largest of all Asian American groups enumerated in the past two census—1980 and 1990 (Barringer, Gardner, and Levin 1993). From 1980 to 1990, the Chinese American population doubled to 1,645,472. The majority (43%) live in California, and another 17% live in New York (Wong 1995; Braun and Browne 1998).

Japanese were the second group of Asian Americans to appear in the census, but their numbers outside Hawaii were similar to those of the Chinese for many years. From 1910 through 1970, Japanese Americans represented over half of the total Asian American population (Barringer, Gardner, and Levin 1993).

Filipinos were the third group of Asian Americans to arrive in the United States. The number of Filipinos grew rapidly at first, to more than 108,000 in 1930, then fluctuated as did the other groups until after 1965, when numbers rose rapidly. The 1970–1980 annual growth rate of 8.2% enabled Filipinos to move into second place among all Asian Americans in terms of numbers (Barringer, Gardner, and Levin 1993).

Asian Indians are the fourth largest group of Asian Americans. Although a few thousand Asian Indians appeared in census reports from time to time, not until 1970 did the Asian Indian population begin to grow rapidly (Barringer, Gardner, and Levin 1993).

Koreans are now the fifth largest Asian American group. By 1970, there were almost 70,000, and since 1970 the growth of the Korean American population has been rapid (Barringer, Gardner, and Levin 1993).

A third group of recent arrivals was the Vietnamese, whose numbers began to rise only in the mid-1970s, after the fall of Saigon and the beginning of the refugee flows. The Vietnamese showed a rapid increase from 1970 to 1980. The Indochinese groups such as the Laotians and Cambodians have also exhibited fast growth rates in the recent decades (Barringer, Gardner, and Levin 1993).

History: Pacific Islanders

In 1980 the census counted 259,566 Pacific Islanders, constituting 7% of the Asian and Pacific Islanders population (Barringer, Gardner, and Levin 1993). In 1990, the 365,024 Pacific Islanders recorded in the U.S. census were 5% of the total Asian and Pacific Islander population. Three large geographical areas identify Pacific Islanders: Polynesia, the largest in area, covers a large triangle, with Hawaii, New Zealand, and Pitcairn Islands forming the three points. The U.S. territory of American Samoa is in Polynesia.

The largest Pacific Islander groups in 1990 were the Hawaiians, Samoans, Guamians, Tongans, and Fijians. Of these groups, Tongans increased the most (183%), and Fijians (146%), second. These groups experienced immigration rates similar to those seen among Asian Americans (Barringer, Gardner, and Levin 1993).

Health-Seeking Process

Asian and Pacific Islander Americans: Symptom Definition

According to the health-seeking model, an individual's symptom definition develops when the degree of discomfort becomes noticeable and acknowledgeable by his or her cultural/ethnic group. If illness receives a cultural stamp, a health care action follows (Chrisman 1977). Chinese medicine, for example, may be divided into three distinct, but related, types: classical Chinese medicine, medicine in contemporary China, and Chinese alternative medicine (Gould-Martin and Ngin 1981). The use of traditional Chinese medicine varies widely according to gender, age, class, region of the United States, generation (first, second, and third), and degree of assimilation to mainstream society.

Classical Chinese medicine is a doctrine based on ancient texts and the principle of the yin and yang. The three most famous texts are the Huang Ti Nei Ching (The Yellow Emperor's Classic of Internal Medicine), the Shang Han Lun (Treatise on Fevers), and the Shen Nung Pen Ts'ao Ching (Shen Nung's Classic Pharmacopeia) (Gould-Martin and Ngin 1981).

Chinese medicine in contemporary China draws ideas from both classical and folk traditions but is a pragmatic and progressive system. The scientific methods of phytochemistry are applied to traditionally prescribed herbs in a search for their active ingredients. Patients preparing for open chest surgery learn ancient breathing exercises. Acupuncture anesthesia is used for cesarean section. Traditional gymnastic exercises are an adjunct treatment for high blood pressure, digestive disorders, and paralysis (Sidel and Sidel 1973). Chinese herb treatment is often given as an alternative to, or in combination with, Western treatment to suit the wishes of the patient and the demands of the disease. Coordinated treatment is carried out under the supervision of professionals from both Western and Chinese medicine (Gould-Martin and Ngin 1981).

Chinese medicine as it is practiced in Chinatowns in the United States is probably closer to folk medicine than to any other system. It is medicine in practice, administered by practitioners who differ widely in background, knowledge, and skill and who are virtually free of the constraints of official supervision (Gould-Martin and Ngin 1981).

The evaluation of symptoms and illness occurs against a background body image: what is in the body, what it looks like, how it functions, and how it is affected by the outside world. For some organs, such as the heart and bowels, a patient has sounds or sensations that help to locate the organ in the body. For others, like the gallbladder, one does not have evidence of the existence of such an organ or of its functioning; as a result, body image is largely a symbolic system with a tenuous connection to anatomy.

Symptoms and disease are most often explained by reference to wind, hot, and cold. A diagnosis of fright may be used to explain why a child is listless, cries at night, refuses food, or has a slight fever. Although this is often a problem related to magic in Asia, in America fright is treated by giving the child "protect-infant-pill," a patent medicine readily available in herb shops and Chinese grocery stores (Gould-Martin and Ngin 1981).

The recommended treatment for a symptom or even the diagnostic procedures indicated may deter patients from treatment and cause them to tolerate their symptoms. Some Chinese are afraid of blood loss, hospitalization, and surgery. Many older people regard the hospital as a place to die, and they confirm that view by waiting until the point of death to go there. The association of the hospital with surgery and death as well as the problems of cost, language, and food all contribute to the practice of delaying hospitalization (Gould-Martin and Ngin 1981).

In traditional Hawaiian culture, illness and other misfortunes are thought to be caused by an imbalance of *mana* (energy that permeates and links all things) or loss of *pono* (rightness or proper order). Dreams are also considered important sources of information, used to solve problems and to forecast events and behaviors (Braun and Browne 1998:269).

Asian Americans: Treatment Actions

The types and sources of treatment actions among Asian Americans are likely to vary according to gender, age, class, region of the United States, generational level, and degree of assimilation to mainstream society. In the United States, as noted earlier, most ethnic groups have the option of selecting from a variety of sources such as (1) formal health professionals; (2) licensed health practitioners; (3) alternative or native health practitioners; (4) lay consultation; and (5) self.

Home preventive treatment, for example, is performed by Chinese Americans as a matter of routine: in hot weather people drink cooling teas and eat more "cold" and cooling foods; in cold weather they consume tonics in the form of soups and special dishes with herbs such as chicken or pork cooked with herbs, dragon eye, and red dates. Other "hot" foods include broccoli, rice wine, liver, mushrooms, ginger, black vinegar, peanuts, and any form of pepper. These are usually taken with the evening meal.

People in a naturally "cold" state (i.e., older people, new mothers, or people with a "cold" constitution) are more careful to avoid "cold" things and consume tonics. People may need special foods to help them through certain stages: adolescence, marriage, and pregnancy. Young, active people who are believed to have warmer bodies will be given more cooling teas, made with "cold" foods such as winter melon, watercress, and water chestnuts. This regimen is not a treatment for a specific ailment. Other "cold" foods include bamboo shoots, melon, soybean sprouts, white turnips, seaweed, mustard greens, bok choy, and chrysa-hemum tea (Cattell 1962).

In addition to herbs and plants, Chinese Americans use other products with medicinal and healing properties. Some of these products were used in ancient Europe and are still used today. Other popular traditional Chinese remedies include the following: deer antlers (used to strengthen bones, increase a man's potency, and dispel nightmares), lime calcium (used to clear excessive mucus), turtle shells (used to stimulate weak kidneys and to remove gallstones), snake flesh (eaten as a delicacy to keep eyes healthy and vision clear), and seahorses (pulverized and used to treat gout) (Spector 1985).

Alternative or native practitioners among Asian Americans are numerous. For example, all the major Chinatowns have numerous traditional practitioners, all of them called (in Chinese) "Chinese doctor." A "Chinese doctor" can do one or more of the following: sell herbs, diagnose minor problems from the patient's appearance and history, make pulse diagnosis, perform acupuncture, and set bones. The flood of immigrants, not only Chinese but also Thai, Korean, and Vietnamese, has provided a demand for traditional practitioners (Gould-Martin and Ngin 1981).

Alternative or native practitioners vary greatly in their style and methods. For instance, traditional Chinese methods for the treatment of illness include acupuncture, moxibustion (described later), respiratory therapy, remedial massage, exercises, treatment of fractures and injuries, and herbal medicine. Though all these methods are used in contemporary China, Taiwan, and Hong Kong, only herbal medicine and acupuncture are common in the United States. Religious and magical healing methods, so common in Hong Kong and Taiwan, are not conspicuously present in Mainland China and the United States (Gould-Martin and Ngin 1981).

Typically, the practitioner writes a prescription that the patient fills at an herb shop. A common prescription, consisting of a mixture of drugs of plant, animal, and mineral origin is boiled in a specified amount of water, and the concoction is taken internally. Sometimes practitioners also prescribe patent medicines, particularly those manufactured in China in recent years.

Acupuncture is an umbrella term that includes many techniques such as acupressure, laser acupuncture, scalp acupuncture, Korean hand acupuncture, moxibustion, electro-acupuncture and more (Ulett, Han, and Han 1998:1115). Most acupuncture techniques involve the use of needles with mystic rituals explained by metaphysical concepts derived from ancient practices of traditional Chinese medicine. The procedure consists of puncturing the body to cure disease or relieve pain. The body is punctured with special metal needles at precise points for the treatment of specific symptoms. The most important aspect of the practice of acupuncture is the acquired skill and ability to know precisely where to puncture the skin (Ceniceros and Brown 1998). Nine needles are used in acupuncture, each with a specific purpose. The following is a list of the needles and their purposes:

1. superficial pricking: arrowhead needle;
2. massaging: round needle;
3. knocking or pressing: blunt needle;
4. venous pricking: sharp, three-edge needle;
5. evacuating pus: swordlike needle;
6. rapid pricking: sharp, round needle;
7. puncturing thick muscle: sharp, round needle;
8. puncturing thick muscle: long needle; and
9. treating arthritis: large needle (Spector 1985).

Moxibustion has been practiced for as long as acupuncture. Its purpose too, is to restore the proper balance of yin and yang. Moxibustion is based on the therapeutic value of heat, whereas acupuncture is a cold treatment. Acupuncture is used mainly in diseases in which there is an excess of yin. Moxibustion is performed by heating pulverized wormwood and applying this concoction directly to the skin over certain specific sites. Moxibustion is believed to be most useful during the period of labor and delivery, if applied properly (Spector 1985). Alternative therapeutic practices and native health practitioners play an important role in the Asian American community.

Conclusion

This section highlights the significant health beliefs and practices among Asian and Pacific Islander Americans. Although there is little documented research on all the various Asian American and Pacific Islander groups, this section uses research studies primarily among Chinese Americans, Japanese Americans, and Hawaiians. Researchers who are concerned with improving our knowledge of the Asian and Pacific Islander American health issues should sample more Asian and Pacific Islander American populations and support a thorough collection and analysis of Asian and Pacific Islander American health data (Braun and Browne 1998).

This brief review of the health beliefs and treatment actions in the context of Asian and Pacific Islander American cultures reflects a broader understanding of the factors that influence their health action (Bailey 1991; Saunders 1954). Moreover, the cultural-historical analysis of Asian and Pacific Islander American traditional health beliefs and treatment actions provides a special insight regarding the cultural bond an individual may develop toward his or her health beliefs and treatment actions.

NATIVE AMERICANS AND ALASKAN NATIVES

Native American and Alaskan Native Culture and Sociodemographics

This section highlights the significant health issues associated with Native Americans and Alaskan Natives. Due to the lack of cultural health data about each Native American and Alaskan Native tribe or nation, this section summarizes the major points of interest about the traditional Native American and Alaskan Native health beliefs and treatment actions. To reiterate, Native American and Alaskan Native health beliefs and treatment actions are likely to vary according to gender, age, class, region of the United States, and degree of assimilation to mainstream society.

Presently, there are approximately 500 federally recognized American Indian tribes in the United States. In 1990, the only tribes with more than 100,000 persons were the Cherokee, Navajo, Chippewa, and Sioux. Approximately 16% of all Indians reported themselves as Cherokee, 12% as Navajo, and 6% each as Chippewa and Sioux (U.S. Department of Commerce 1993). The Choctaw, Pueblo, and Apache had populations of at least 50,000 persons. The Choctaw accounted for 4% of the Native American population. The Iroquois Confederacy, Lumbee, and Creek all had 43,000 or more persons. The 1990 census showed that fourteen tribes had a population between 10,000 and 21,000 persons. Most tribes had populations of less than 10,000 (U.S. Department of Commerce 1993).

Native Americans and Alaskan Natives live predominantly in 26 states, with most residing in the western part of the country as a result of forced westward migration. Although many Indians remain on reservations and in rural areas, just as many of them live in cities, especially those on the West Coast. Oklahoma,

Arizona, California, New Mexico, and Alaska have the largest numbers of Native Americans (Spector 1985).

Additional sociodemographics of importance are migration patterns and the percentage of elders. Approximately 54% of Native Americans and Alaskan Natives have migrated from reservations to urban areas, primarily for economic opportunity. Moreover, the Native American and Alaskan Native elders make up approximately 6% of the Native American and Alaskan Native population and are the fastest growing ethnic population (Rousseau 1995:83).

The Native American family unit is an essential component to an individual's total health. Family is a kinship-structured unit, related to blood, marriage, cohabitation, or adoption. It is sustained through constant physical and psychosocial contact through interacting and carrying out life functions (Miller 1980; Sobralske 1985). These ties usually play an important role in the individual's health beliefs and treatment actions.

History: Native American and Alaskan Native

The earliest accounts of Native Americans and Alaskan Natives in North America date approximately 30,000 years ago. Archaeological evidence indicates that a small number of Native American hunting groups filtered gradually into North America (Spector 1985; Harwood 1981; Young 1994). Native Americans and Alaskan Natives began to diversify as they adapted to new conditions. Despite the numerous disruptions and dislocations from their native habits, Native Americans' and Alaskan Natives' ancient cultural traits have survived for centuries, such as the predominance of tribal or group councils, tribal languages, hunting ceremonialism, and a deeply spiritual religious and health belief system (Hultkrantz 1992; Spector 1985; Harwood 1981; Young 1994).

Health-Seeking Process

Native American and Alaskan Native Symptom Definition

According to the health care-seeking model, an individual's symptom definition develops when the degree of discomfort becomes noticeable and acknowledgeable by his or her cultural group. If illness receives a cultural stamp, then a health care action follows (Chrisman 1977). Many Native Americans with traditional orientations believe there is a reason for every sickness or pain. They believe that it is a price that is being paid, either for something that happened in the past or for something that will happen in the future. In spite of this conviction, a sick person must still be cared for. Everything is seen as being the result of something else, and this cause-and-effect relationship creates an eternal chain. Native Americans do not subscribe to the germ theory of modern medicine. Illness is something that must be. Even the person who is experiencing the illness may not realize the reason for its occurrence, but it may be the best possible price to pay for the past or future (Spector 1985).

According to Navajo belief system (southwest Native American), disease may be contracted by five basic methods:

1. soul loss;
2. intrusive object;
3. spirit possession;
4. breach of taboo; and
5. witchcraft (Kunitz and Levy 1981; Spector 1985).

The notion of soul loss is not a major means by which specific diseases are caused, yet there is reason to believe that the concept is very important to Native Americans. The soul, or wind, as it is most often called, enters the body soon after birth and forms the individual's basic personality. At death, the soul leaves the body and proceeds to the afterworld. Faintness and suffocation are signs that the wind-soul is leaving the body and signal the final stage of an illness (Kunitz and Levy 1981).

In addition, some form of breach of taboo is the most frequently reported kind of diagnosis among the Navajo. Breach of taboo is not only the commission of prohibited acts but also coming into contact with a "dangerous" object. The responsibility for breaking a taboo may lie with someone other than the afflicted. Thus, a pregnant woman may breach a taboo and cause her child to become ill later in life (Kunitz and Levy 1981).

Native American and Alaskan Native Treatment Actions

There are variations in healing procedure from tribe to tribe and in different culture areas. However, some methods are nearly universal. For instance, the traditional healer of Native American is the medicine man, and they have maintained their faith in him over the ages. He is a person wise in the ways of the land and of nature. He knows well the interrelationships of human beings, the earth, and the universe. He knows the ways of the plants and animals, the sun, the moon, and the stars. The medicine man takes his time to determine the cause and treatment of an illness and then the proper treatment. In order to determine the cause and treatment of an illness, he performs special ceremonies that may take up to several days (Vogel 1970).

There is also the diagnostician. The function of the diagnostician is first to determine the cause of the illness and then to recommend the treatment, that is, the type of chant that will be effective and the medicine man who can best do it. The diagnostician may suggest one of three types of divination: motion in the hand (the most common form and often practiced by women), stargazing (prayers to the star spirit asking it to show him the cause of the illness), and listening (cause of the illness is determined by the sound that is heard) (Spector 1991).

Native Americans and Alaskan Natives also rely upon the extensive use of herbal remedies. There are specific rituals to be followed when herbs are utilized and gathered. Each plant is picked to be dried for later use. No plant is picked unless it is the proper one, and only enough plants are picked to meet the needs of the patient. Timing is crucial, and procedures are followed (Spector 1991).

Various plants are thought to be good for treating a large variety of symptoms. Native Americans and Alaskan Natives who have a knowledge of these plants and who are able to obtain them utilize them much as the general population uses aspirin (Harwood 1981).

For example, the native medicines commonly included leaves, flowers, fruits, barks, seeds, or roots used for their astringent effect in diarrhea and hemorrhage. In several tribes, the root bark of dogwood is a diarrhea remedy, while the dried bark of sweet gum, often mixed with red-oak bark, is used against dysentery (Harwood 1981).

Numerous herbal remedies were used by Native Americans to promote diuresis. Aztec remedies for dysuria included atoll, a mixture of raw ground maize and water, which was a panacea for a myriad of ills. The leaves of *ixyayaual* or mountain balm and the ground root of a gourd vine are called *oquichpatli*, which was mixed with grass and rubber for a suppository (Vogel 1970). These herbal remedies are just a few examples of the type of herbal remedies used by Native American and Alaskan Natives.

Conclusion

This section highlights the significant health beliefs and treatment actions among Native Americans and Alaskan Natives. Current health research has not documented thoroughly the health beliefs and treatment actions of the numerous Native American and Alaskan Native tribes. Today, Native Americans and Alaskan Natives are faced with a number of health-related issues. Many of the old ways of diagnosing and treating illness have been modified and changed. Yet it is still important to understand the framework of Native Americans' and Alaskan Natives' traditional health beliefs and treatment actions in order for any intervention to occur.

POST-EVALUATION QUESTIONS

1. Now that you are aware of different health beliefs and treatment actions of the U.S. ethnic minority populations, how can you be more effective in researching health care issues?

2. How can health care professionals incorporate an understanding of an ethnic groups' health beliefs into their practice?

3. How can a public health administrator use this information when planning a public health program?

REFERENCES

Abril, I.F. 1977. "Mexican American Folk Beliefs: How They Affect Health Care." *The American Journal of Maternal Child Nursing* (May/June): 168–173.

Ailinger, R. L. 1985. "Beliefs about Treatment of Hypertension among Hispanic Older Persons." *Topics in Clinical Nursing* 7: 26–31.

Bailey, Eric. 1991a. "Hypertension: An Ethnomedical Analysis of Detroit African American Treatment Patterns." *Human Organization* 50: 287–296.

———. 1991b. *Urban African American Health Care*. Lanham, MD: University Press of America.

———. 1994. "The Health Status of African Americans in Indianapolis." *Journal of the National Medical Association* 86: 853-856.

Barringer, Herbert, Robert Gardner, and Michael Levin. 1993. *Asians and Pacific Islanders in the United States*. New York: Russell Sage Foundation.

Beals, R. L. 1946. *Cheran: A Sierra Tarascan Village*. Publications of the Institute of Social Anthropology. Smithsonian Institution 2: I-225.

Blaisdell, Richard. 1989 "Historical and Cultural Aspects of Native Hawaiian Health." *Social Process in Hawaii* 32: 1–21.

———. 1993 "The Health Status of the Kanak Maoli." *Asian American and Pacific Islander Journal of Health* 1:116–160.

Braun, Kathryn, and Colette Browne. 1998. "Perceptions of Dementia, Caregiving, and Help Seeking among Asian and Pacific Islander Americans." *Health and Social Work* 23:262–274.

Cattell, Stuart. 1962. *Health, Welfare an Social Organization in Chinatown, New York City*. New York: Community Service Society.

Ceniceros, Salvador, and George Brown. 1998. "Acupuncture: A Review of its History, Theories, and Indications." *Southern Medical Journal* 91: 1121–1125.

Chan, Chun-Wai, and J. Change. 1976. "The Role of Chinese Medicine in New York City's Chinatown." *American Journal of Chinese Medicine* 4:31–45, 129–146.

Chesney, A.P., B.L. Thompson, A. Guevara. 1980. "Mexican American Folk Medicine: Implications for the Family Physician." *The Journal of Family Practice* 11:4: 567–574.

Chrisman, Noel. 1977. "The Health Seeking Process: An Approach to the Natural History of Illness." *Culture and Medical Psychiatry* 1:351-377.

Clark, M. 1959. *Health in the Mexican American Culture*. Berkeley: University of California Press.

Cockerham, William. 1986. *Medical Sociology*. Englewood Cliffs, NJ.: Prentice-Hall.

Coulehan, J.L. 1976. "Navajo Indian Medicine: A Dimension in Healing." *Pharos* 39: 93-96.

Croizier, Ralph. 1968. *Traditional Medicine in Modern China*. Cambridge: Harvard University Press.

Currier, Richard. 1966. "The Hot-Cold Syndrome and Symbolic Balance in Mexican and Spanish American Folk Medicine." *Ethnology* 5: 251-263.

Edgerton, Robert, M. Karno, and I. Fernandez. 1970. "Curanderismo in the Metropolis." *American Journal of Psychotherapy* 24: 124–134.

Foster, George. 1953. "Relationship between Spanish and Spanish American Folk Medicine." *Journal of American Folklore* 66: 201–218.

———. 1987. "On the Origin of Humoral Medicine in Latin America." *Medical Anthropology Quarterly* 1: 355-393.

Foster, George and Barbara Anderson. 1978. *Medical Anthropology*. New York: Alfred A. Knopf

Fuchs, M., and R. Bashur. 1975. "Use of Traditional Indian Medicine among Urban Native Americans." *Medical Care* 13: 915–927.

Gould-Martin, K., and C. Ngin. 1981. "Chinese Americans." In *Ethnicity and Medical Care*. A. Harwood, ed. Pp. 130–171. Cambridge: Harvard University Press.

Harwood, Alan. 1971. "The Hot-Cold Theory of Disease." *Journal of the American Medical Association* 216:1153–1158.

———. 1981. *Ethnicity and Medical Care*. Cambridge: Harvard University Press.

Hill, Carole. 1976. "Folk Medical Belief System in the American South: Some Practical Considerations." *Southern Medicine*. December: 11-17.

Hostetter, T. 1984. "Entering a Native American Community to Assess Nurses' Continuing Education Needs in the Area of Mental Health." *Journal of Continuing Education in Nursing* 15:188–190.

Hultkrantz, Ake. 1992. *Shamanic Healing and Ritual Drama: Health and Medicine in Native North American Religious Traditions*. New York: The Crossroad Publishing Company.

Ingham, John. 1970. "On Mexican Folk Medicine." *American Anthropologist* 72: 76–87.

Kay, Margarita. 1979. "Health and Illness in a Mexican American Barrio." In *Ethnic Medicine in the Southwest*. E. Spicer, ed. Pp. 99–160. Tucson: University of Arizona Press.

Kiev, Ari. 1968. Curanderismo: *Mexican American Folk Psychiatry*. New York: The Free Press.

Klein, S. 1978. "Susto: The Anthropological Study of Disease of Adaptation." *Social Science and Medicine* 12–23.

Kunitz, Stephen, and J. Levy. 1981. "Navajos." In *Ethnicity and Medical Care*, A Harwood, ed. Pp. 337–396. Cambridge: Harvard University Press.

———. 1983. *Disease Change and Role of Medicine: The Navajo Experience*. Berkeley: University of California Press.

Landy, David. 1977. *Culture, Disease, and Healing*. New York: Macmillan.

Latin American Wave. 1997. "What Is an Hispanic?" Indianapolis: October. P. 6.

Lucero, G. 1975. "Health and Illness in the Chicano Community." Lecture given at Boston College School of Nursing: March.

Madsen, William. 1964. *Mexican Americans of South Texas*. New York: Holt, Rinehart, and Winston.

Mayers, Raymond. 1989. "Use of Folk Medicine by Elderly Mexican American Women." *The Journal of Drug Issues* 19: 283–295.

McFeeley, F. 1949. *"Some Aspects of Folk Curing in the American Southwest."* M.A. Thesis, University of California.

Miller, J. and E. Janosik. 1980. *Family-Focused Care.* New York: McGraw-Hill.

Min, Pyong. 1995. *Asian Americans: Contemporary Trends and Issues.* Thousand Oaks, CA: Sage.

Mindel, Charles and Robert Habenstein. 1981. *Ethnic Families in America: Patterns and Variations. Second Edition.* New York: Elsevier.

Pachter, Lee, Michelle Cloutier, and Bruce Bernstein. 1995. "Ethnomedical (Folk) Remedies for Childhood Asthma in a Mainland Puerto Rican Community." *Archives Pediatric Adolescence Medicine* 149: 982–988.

Padilla, E. 1958. *Up from Puerto Rico.* New York: Columbia University Press.

Randall-David, Elizabeth. 1989. *Strategies for Working with Culturally Diverse Communities and Clients.* Washington DC: Publication No. 0-937821-58-6. U.S. Dept. of Health and Human Services, Association for the Care of Children's Health.

Ripley, G.D. 1986. "Mexican American Folk Remedies: Their Place in Health Care." *Texas Medicine/Folk Medicine* 82: 41–44.

Risser, Amanda, and Lynette Mazur. 1995. "Use of Folk Remedies in a Hispanic Population." *Archives Pediatric Adolescence Medicine* 149: 978–981.

Rivera, George. 1988. "Hispanic Folk Medicine Utilization in Urban Colorado." *Sociology and Social Research* 72: 237–241.

Rosa, Mario. 1988. "Natural Support Systems of Puerto Ricans: A Key Dimension for Well-Being." *Health and Social Work* 13: 181–190.

Rousseau, Paul. 1995. "Native-American Elders: Health Care Status." *Clinics in Geriatric Medicine* 11: 83–95.

Rubel, Arthur. 1960. "Concepts of Disease in Mexican American Culture." *American Anthropologist* 62: 795–815.

———. 1977. "The Epidemiology of a Folk Illness: Susto in Hispanic America." In *Culture, Disease, and Healing: Studies in Medical Anthropology.* D. Landy, ed. Pp: 119–128. New York: Macmillan.

Saunders, L. 1954. *Cultural Differences in Medical Care.* New York: Russell Sage.

Sidel, Victor and Ruth Sidel. 1984. *Reforming Medicine: Lessons of the Last Quarter Century.* New York: Pantheon Books.

Simmen, E. 1972. *Pain and Promise: The Chicano Today.* New York: New American Library.

Sobralske, Mary. 1985. "Perceptions of Health: Navajo Indians." *Topics in Clinical Nursing* 7: 32–39.

Spector, Rachel. 1985. "Health and Illness in the Native American Community." In *Cultural Diversity and Health Care.* R. Spector, ed. Pp. 235–257. New York: Appleton-Century Crofts.

———. 1991. *Cultural Diversity and Health Care.* New York: Appleton-Century Crofts.

Spicer, Edward. 1979. *Ethnic Medicine in the Southwest*. Tucson: University of Arizona Press.

Stern, Michael. 1993. "Cardiovascular and Other Chronic Diseases among Mexican Americans: The Emerging Picture." *Ethnicity and Disease* 3: 7–10.

Steward, J.H. 1956. *People of Puerto Rico: A Study in Social Anthropology*. Urbana, IL: University of Illinois Press.

Sullivan, Louis. 1992. "Keynote Address" at the Surgeon General's National Workshop on Hispanic/Latino Health Workshop. September. Washington, DC.

Topley, Marjorie. 1970. "Chinese Traditional Ideas and the Treatment of Disease: Two Examples from Hong Kong." *Man* 5:421–437.

Ulett, George, Jisheng Han, and Songpin Han. 1998. "Traditional and Evidence-Based Acupuncture: History, Mechanisms, and Present Status." *Southern Medical Journal* 91: 1115–1120.

U.S. Department of Commerce. 1993a. *We the American Asians*. Economics and Statistics Administration. Bureau of Census.

———. 1993b. *We the First Americans*. Economics and Statistics Administration. Bureau of Census.

———. 1993c. *We the American Hispanics*. Economics and Statistics Administration. Bureau of Census.

U.S. Department of Health and Human Services. 1985. *Black & Minority Health: The Secretary Task Force on Minority Health*. Washington, DC: U.S. Government Printing Office.

U.S. Department of Health and Human Services. 1997. *Health United States 1996-97 and Injury Chartbook*. National Center for Health Statistics. Washington, DC: U.S. Government Printing Office. DHHS Publication No. 97-1232.

Vazquez, Andrew, and Aurora Ramirez-Krodel. 1989. *America's Hispanic Heritage: An Overview of Hispanics in the United States*. Ann Arbor. University of Michigan Press.

Vogel, Virgil. 1970 *American Indian Medicine*. Norman: University of Oklahoma Press.

Warren, Rueben. 1992. "Health Education and Black Health Status." In *Health Issues in the Black Community*. R. Braithwaite and S. Taylor, eds. Pp. 241–254. San Francisco: Jossey Bass.

Wong, M.G. 1995 "Chinese Americans." In *Asian Americans: Contemporary Trends and Issues*. P.G. Minn, ed. Pp. 58–94. Thousand Oaks, CA: Sage.

Young, T. Kue. 1994. *The Health of Native Americans: Toward a Biocultural Epidemiology*. New York: Oxford University Press.

Zane, N., D. Takeuchi, and K. Young. 1994. *Confronting Critical Health Issues of Asian and Pacific Islander Americans*. Thousand Oaks, CA: Sage.

WEB SITES OF SIGNIFICANCE

Centers for Disease Control and Prevention

http://www.cdc.gov/

National Institutes of Health

http://www.nih.gov/

Office of the Associate Director for Minority Health

http://www.cdc.gov/od/admh/plan.htm/

Office of Minority Health Resource Center

http://www.omhrc.gov/

U.S. Department of Health and Human Services

http://www.os.dhhs.gov/

Part II

African American Health Care

African American health care is discussed in three chapters. Chapter 3 concentrates on the culture of African Americans and the sociocultural health issues related to the African American population. Chapter 4 focuses on the major diseases associated with African Americans and the most recent documented research studies investigating African American cultural health care issues. Finally, Chapter 5 discusses African Americans' alternative medical practices in the context of their history, current health and illness situations, and treatment actions. This section on African American health care is subdivided into three separate chapters primarily because it is the most effective approach to show how medical anthropology examines current health issues among African Americans.

Chapter 3

African American Health Care:
A Cultural Relativistic Perspective

CRITICAL THINKING QUESTIONS

1. Is it necessary to examine African American health from a new perspective?

2. Are there advantages in viewing African American health from a cultural relativistic perspective?

3. What can the health care professional learn from adopting the cultural relativistic perspective?

INTRODUCTION

Medical anthropologists are trained to view the health status of each individual and population from a biopsychosociocultural perspective. As stated in Chapter 1, our approach is holistic; that is, medical anthropologists believe that all factors contribute to the well-being or sickness of a person/population. In order to understand how this biopsychosociocultural, or holistic, approach applies to African Americans, this chapter examines the cultural component of the biopsychosociocultural model by:

1. highlighting the culture of African Americans and then discussing how culture relates to African American health;
2. examining the major sociodemographics associated with the African American population and the cultural patterns that are reflected in these sociodemographic patterns;
3. examining psychosocial issues, such as religion and caregiving, and how these factors relate to African American health; and
4. examining the major cultural historical health issues that may have had an impact on the health-seeking process of the African American population.

For many medical anthropologists, one of the key factors is culture. When working with the African American population, understanding African American culture is a key to any health assessment, health care intervention, and health care policy.

AFRICAN AMERICAN CULTURE

This book defines culture as "a people who share a common history, place of origin, language, food preferences, spirituality, health beliefs, and values that engender a sense of exclusiveness and self-awareness of being a member of this ethnic group." Although African Americans demonstrate and express African American culture differently and similarly from one region of the United States to another or from one community to another, there is one distinctive commonality: the African American family.

Much has been written about the African American family, and one particular element is certain. The African American family as a unit has a historical continuity that began not with the American experience but in Africa long before the intrusion of Europe into that continent.

As early as the 1500s and 1600s, the descendants of African Americans (West Africans) were forcibly transported to South America, the Caribbean, and North America. In the process of adapting to the new environments, these West Africans merged their cultural traditions with European and Native American traditions. Although some of the cultural traditions have changed or been *Americanized*, the family unit remains constant.

The structural characteristics of the African American family today include:

1.   a bilateral orientation—an equal recognition of the male and female line of descent but with an emphasis favoring the mother's kin;
2.   extended kin groups existing in a social environment in which primary-type relations are extended into the larger community;
3.   emphasis on respect for elders; and
4.   a high value placed on children and motherhood. (Aschenbrenner 1973; Stack 1974)

In addition to these structural characteristics, there are some other values and characteristics of African American families:

1.   a high value of family and individual moral "strength" as a human quality;
2.   an emphasis on family occasions and rituals; and
3.   strong belief in spiritualism (Aschenbrenner 1973; Stack 1974).

With regard to specific cultural patterns, there have been a number of generally agreed upon cultural traits associated with African Americans. The following list is not an exclusive list, nor does it provide all the traits of African

Americans, it is a baseline of cultural traits or patterns that have been associated with African Americans.

- Respect toward elders.
- Reliance upon extended familial network for social, economic, and health care issues.
- Strong orientation toward religious beliefs, activities, and organizations.
- Outwardly expressed emotions.
- Emphasis in nurturing children and participating in many rites of passages.
- Preference for group activities as opposed to individual activities.
- Preference for oral communication and oral history to share news and information.
- Admiration of art, dance, and music.
- Preference for a bilateral kinship system—trace descent equally through males and females.
- Preference for women and men sharing roles and responsibilities.

The African American culture list highlights the importance of culture to its people and also emphasizes how the attributes of culture relate to African American health care issues.

Culture is a learned process. African Americans learn certain health beliefs and practices from their extended familial network. When a health care crisis occurs, African Americans tend to seek health care information from their extended familial network or a lay health professional first, then opt for professional care.

Culture is transmitted by symbols verbally and nonverbally. African Americans are acutely aware of nonverbal body language that indicates that a health care provider is comfortable or not comfortable in treating an African American person. If the African American patient perceives the nonverbal language as positive, he or she will most likely return for care. However, if the African American patient perceives the nonverbal body language as negative, he or she will most likely not return for care and not adhere to the prescribed regimen.

Culture is integrated. Like all Americans, African Americans are connected to the social, economic, political, and health care fabric of our society. Yet once an economic or health care crisis occurs in U.S. society, African Americans often are affected first primarily because a third of the population are considered the working poor.

Culture adds meaning to reality. African Americans respect and honor those who train, graduate, and serve in the health professional fields. Often, African American health care professionals feel a commitment to serve their community. Because of the low numbers of African American physicians and health care specialists, African Americans frequently choose to work in underserved, minority communities as opposed to communities with relatively low numbers of minorities. African Americans' commitment to work and to serve those who are underserved adds meaning to their profession of the health care field.

Culture is differently shared. African Americans perceive health and the health care system differently. Although African Americans have many common traits and patterns, there remains a high degree of diversity within the African American population. For instance, intragenerational health care issues differ among African Americans as they relate to perceptions of the health care system and health belief system. Additional sociodemographic factors such as gender, region of the country, income level, and educational level may also cause differing perceptions of health care issues in the African American population.

Culture is adaptive. Traditionally, African Americans have always had to adapt to social, economic, political, and health care barriers to mainstream society. Whether the barriers are actual or perceived, African Americans learn alternative patterns of utilizing the local health care system. Chapter 5 discusses a variety of alternative medical practices among African Americans.

AFRICAN AMERICAN SOCIODEMOGRAPHICS

To better understand the relationship between culture and health care issues associated with the African American population, we must examine the current social, economic, and demographic data from the U.S. Census. Although recently there has been much discussion on the lack of reporting and inaccuracy of the U.S. Census data and the fact that many African Americans are very skeptical of any governmental data agency, the sociodemographic data show some very intriguing and positive trends associated with the African American population. The following are highlighted sociodemographic trends as reported by the U.S. Census Bureau (1998):

- On October 1, 1996, there were an estimated 33.7 million African Americans in the United States, constituting 12.7% of the total population. Their median age was 29.4 years.
- It's projected that the African American population will grow more than twice as fast as the white population between 1995 and 2050. The African American population would increase by 2 million by 2000, 7 million by 2010, and 17 million by 2030. By the middle of the next century, the African American population would nearly double its present size to 61 million.
- After 2016, more African Americans than non-Hispanic whites are expected to be added to the U.S. population each year.
- The African American population is young, with an estimated median age on November 1, 1997, of 29.8 years, nearly 8 years younger than the median for the non-Hispanic white population.

- In 1996, 53% of African Americans lived in the South, making up 19% of that region's population. Nationwide, 55% resided in the central cities of metropolitan areas.

- Five states had more than 2 million African American residents on July 1, 1996: New York (3.2 million), California (2.4 million), Texas (2.3 million), Florida (2.2 million), and Georgia (2.1 million).

- The ten counties with the most African American residents on July 1, 1996, were Cook, Illinois (1.4 million), Los Angeles, (1.0 million), Kings, New York (900,000), Wayne, Michigan. (900,000), Philadelphia, (600,000), Harris, Texas (600,000), Bronx, New York (500,000), Queens, New York (500,000), Dade, Florida (400,000), and Baltimore City, Maryland (400,000).

- In 1997, 6% of blacks (2.0 million) were foreign-born.

- In 1996, there were 8.1 million African American families, 46% of them married-couple families. The majority of African American families (57%) had children. Families with children averaged two children apiece.

- Forty-one percent of African American men and 37% of women aged fifteen and over were married in 1996.

- About one in eight African American children under eighteen years age lived in the home of their grandparents in 1995, compared with 1 in 25 white children. About one-third of African American children lived with both parents.

- In 1996, African American households had a median income of $23,482 statistically unchanged from 1995. Meanwhile, per capita income for African Americans, adjusted for inflation, increased 5.2% from 1995 to 1996, to $11,899.

- African American households were the only racial or ethnic group to experience an increase in real median income between 1993 and 1994. Their median income rose from $20,032 to $21,027, an increase of 5.0%, the first significant annual increase among African Americans in income since 1989.

- In 1996, the poverty rate for African Americans was 28.4%, unchanged from 1995.

- Between 1993 and 1994, poverty rates dropped for African Americans (from 33.1% to 30.6%) and for whites (from 12.2% to 11.7%).

- In 1996, 16% of African American men and 22% of African American women aged sixteen and over worked in managerial and professional specialty jobs (e.g., engineers, dentists, teachers, lawyers, and reporters).

- The number of African American-owned businesses in the United States increased 46%, from 424,165 to 620,912, between 1987 and 1992. Receipts for these firms increased by 63% during the five-year span, from $19.8 billion to $32.2 billion. The total number of all the nation's firms increased 26% from 13.7 million in 1987 to 17.3 million in 1992. Their receipts grew 67%, from $2 trillion to $3 trillion.

- In 1996, 74% of the nation's African Americans aged 25 and over had at least a high school diploma. This proportion is up from 1980, when 51% had attained at least a high school diploma. The growth was similar for African American males and females.

- In 1997, 86% of African Americans ages 25 to 29 were high school graduates.

- The gap in high school completion between African Americans and whites narrowed in the 25-to-29 year-old age group over the past decade (1980s) to the point where there was no statistical difference in 1997.

- In 1996, 14% of the nation's African Americans aged 25 and over had earned at least a bachelor's degree, up from 8%, respectively in 1980.

- African American preschoolers were less likely to be cared for by nonrelatives or in organized child care facilities than white preschoolers (48% compared to 54%).

- In 1993, about four in ten African American preschoolers were cared for by grandparents or other relatives besides their fathers while their mothers worked, compared to only about two in ten white children. Care by grandparents was especially important to African American families, accounting for one-fifth of all arrangements used for preschoolers. (U.S. Census Bureau: Public Information Office, January 26, 1998, January 31, 1997, and February 5, 1996).

To summarize, the sociodemographics show that the African American population will continue to increase in the future (actually doubling by the middle of the next century), will improve their economic, income, and educational attainments, will continue to have children in their families (average two apiece), and, most importantly, will continue to have extended family members (grandparents and others) to assist in raising children. These sociodemographic trends present an excellent example of the interrelationship of cultural patterns with sociodemographic data. African American culture emphasizing respect toward elders, reliance upon extended familial network, and the nurturing of children, has a direct impact on such issues as who often cares for the African American preschooler; the type of flexible household structure, depending on the family's income level; and the pattern of seeking health care for the individual African American.

AFRICAN AMERICAN PSYCHOSOCIAL ISSUES

Another important factor to the biopsychosociocultural model is the psychosocial component. For the purpose of our discussion, this book refers to psychosocial factors in a broad-based sense, encompassing such issues as mental health, religiosity, and spirituality. In particular, mental health and religiosity play a significant role in the well-being of the African American population.

Mental Health

Good mental health refers not only to freedom from major depression or psychiatric disorders but, more importantly, to the ability to cope effectively with life's daily stresses and feel good about one's overall physical, social, and spiritual well-being (Neighbors 1991). Yet, at least one of every five adults has a dysfunction in one mental health domain or another. Mental health issues include depression, anxiety, posttraumatic stress, eating disorders, and suicide.

The prevalence of mental health disorders among African Americans is similar to that of U.S. population as a whole, but cultural beliefs and cultural health-seeking patterns may keep many African Americans with mental health disorders from seeking or receiving diagnosis, treatment, and rehabilitation (National Mental Health Association 1994). In fact, at a 1994 congressional briefing on the recognition and treatment of mental illnesses in the African American community held June 22 in Washington, DC, the Congressional Black Caucus, the National Mental Health Association, and the National Institute on Mental Health cited that a number of barriers between the community and practitioners which have prevented effective understanding and intervention.

For example, many African Americans with mental disorders who do seek help are not accurately diagnosed because the frequency with which they report some symptoms differs from that in the overall U.S. population or because colloquial descriptions of symptoms may not be consistent with mental health practitioners' understanding of diagnostic criteria (National Mental Health Association 1994). Additionally, myths such as the belief that if one is oppressed, it makes sense to be depressed and that mental illnesses are not treatable or not worth treating hinders African Americans from being properly treated.

To determine whether the myths and the pattern of seeking care for mental health disorders existed in the African American community, McMiller and Weisz (1996) focused on families of children (including adolescents) who had been admitted to care in a mental health clinic. The sample of 192 included 123 boys and 69 girls; the age range was from seven through seventeen years. Sixty-three percent were European American, 17% African American, and 20% were Latino.

McMiller and Weisz (1996) found that European American parents were likely to make their initial contact with professionals and agencies, whereas African American and Latino parents were especially likely to make their initial contact with family and community members, not with professionals or agency personnel. Specifically, more than two-thirds of African American and Latino parents sought help initially from family and community contacts; and a majority of all preclinic contacts in these groups were nonprofessional and non-agency-related. This pattern stands in contrast to that of the European American parents, for whom a majority of first contacts and a majority of total contacts were with professionals and agencies (McMiller and Weisz 1996: 1092).

McMiller and Weisz (1996) contend that their findings also carry implications for the design of community mental health outreach efforts. The low level of professional and agency contact seen among African American and Latino families suggests that efforts by clinics and mental health program planners to expand their outreach to minority groups by notifying other agencies and professionals of their services may be incomplete at best. Instead, McMiller and Weisz (1996) suggest that their findings point to the need to reach more deeply into ethnic communities, extending beyond the professional level to reach those community leaders and family members most likely to be sought out by troubled minority group families seeking help for their children.

Religion and Spirituality

The links between religious involvement and personal well-being have received increasing attention from scholars (Schumaker 1992; Levin 1996 and et al. 1997). Ellison (1995) states that although the empirical evidence is not unequivocal, the findings to date suggest that various aspects of religious practice, affiliation, and belief have beneficial implications for mental health.

In fact, research in the epidemiology of religion has increased the validity of religion and spirituality as topics for still further medical research (Levin et al. 1997). The National Institutes of Health (NIH) funded research investigating religion as a determinant of physical and mental health in 1995 and sponsored a conference titled, "Methodological Approaches to the Study of Religion, Health, and Aging" and "Spiritual Assessment in Health Care Settings" (Levin et al. 1997: 792).

The church, one of the symbols for religious involvement, has long been one of the major social and cultural institutions that define how people should see themselves and direct their behavior (Berry and Blassingame 1982). Taylor and Chatters (1991) emphasizes that the teachings of the church regarding human nature and human relationships may foster either mentally healthy attitudes or destructive, neurotic attitudes in its members. Inevitably, a church teaches its members, either directly or indirectly, how to deal with aggression, anger, pride, sexuality, competition, social relations, child-raising, and marital relations (Taylor and Chatters 1991).

Within the African American community, the significance of African American church to community life may be attributed, in part, to their position as one of the few indigenous institutions in African American communities that are built, financed, and controlled by African Americans. Moreover, African American churches serve as an outlet for social expression, a forum for the discussion of political and social issues, and a training ground for potential community leaders (Chatters et al. 1998; Neighbors et al. 1998; and McRae et al. 1998).

In 1991, Taylor and Chatters reported the results from a National Survey on Black Americans (N = 2,094) with regard to religious affiliations among African Americans. Taylor and Chatters (1991) found the following results:

1.   Forty different religious affiliations were reported;

2. One-half of the respondents indicated that they were Baptist (52.1%);
3. Eleven percent were Methodist;
4. Six percent were Roman Catholic;
5. Three percent were Holiness;
6. Two percent were Jehovah's Witness;
7. Fifteen percent identified one or more of the 35 remaining denominations;
8. One out of ten respondents indicated no religious preference; and
9. Eight respondents indicated that they were either atheist or agnostic (Taylor and Chatter 1991: 108).

In a study to examine the significance of religiosity and health outcomes among African Americans, Picot et al. (1997) conducted face-to-face interviews of 136 African Americans and 255 European American caregivers of community-dwelling elders. Results revealed that African American caregivers perceived higher levels of rewards from participating in religious services than did European American caregivers. Additionally, the relationship between race and perceived rewards was mediated by comfort from religion and prayer. African Americans are taught to depend on a supreme being, the Lord, and take their burdens to the Lord and leave them there (Picot et al. 1997). Picot et al. (1997) contend that these findings suggest a need for health care providers to assess the importance of religious beliefs and health outcomes among all groups, particularly the effects within the African American population.

CULTURAL HISTORICAL FACTORS

Another component to the comprehensive, biopsychosociocultural approach to health is cultural history. The cultural historical approach helps us to better understand issues such as

1. African Americans' past health-seeking process;
2. African Americans' current perceptions of the national and local health care system;
3. African Americans' lack of participation in clinical trials; and
4. African Americans' alternative medical practices.

In addition, this approach examines the sensitive, ethical health care issues that are often associated with the African American population (Bailey 1994).

The significance of the cultural historical approach can best be illustrated in the following articles. In an article entitled, "African American Suspicion of the HealthCare System Is Justified: What Do We Do about It?" Dula (1994) uses historical and contemporary examples of health care issues that contributed to the mistrust and suspicion that many African Americans believe about the U.S. health care system. According to Dula (1994), three major factors contribute to the distrust: (1) real abuses in experimentation, sickle cell screening, and involuntary sterilization, (2) beliefs that the government is responsible for the AIDS epidemic, and (3) real fears and anxieties concerning future medical abuses.

The first factor of distrust involves real abuses in experimentation. Historically, the U.S. health care system has used some unethical medical procedures on the African American population. Dula (1994) highlights six sources of distrust:

1. slaves as experimental and teaching material;
2. the Tuskegee experiment: a symbol of mistrust;
3. sickle cell screening and good intentions;
4. involuntary sterilization;
5. attitudes about AIDS: a genocidal plot; and
6. the violence initiative: a gene for aggression and young black males.

Each of these beliefs and documented incidents contributed significantly to the feeling of distrust among many African Americans.

Suspicion of the medical system in the United States has its origin in slavery medical practices. Dula (1994) states that slaves were sources for medical experimentation and research for doctors, they were instructional material for medical students, and enslaved albinos and Siamese twins were displayed as freaks and sports at medical society meetings. African Americans contributed to scientific progress, usually without consent or benefit to themselves and sometimes without benefit even to science (Dula 1994: 348).

Another cultural historical case is the Tuskegee experiment. Dula (1994) states that the Tuskegee experiment (1932)—in which 400 African American men participated in a government-sponsored study to find the effects of untreated syphilis—was the ultimate proof that European American health policymakers, indeed, deserved the mistrust. Jones (1981) and Dalton (1989) support Dula's claim. Thomas and Quinn (1991), who stated the following, also support Dula: "The history of the Tuskegee Syphilis Study, with its failure to educate the participants and treat them adequately, helped to lay the foundation for Blacks' pervasive sense of distrust of public health authorities today" (1499).

Additional cases of mistrust were sickle-cell screening (confusion regarding differences between carriers and those suffering from the disease), involuntary sterilization (perception that family planning clinics practice sterilization among public-assisted African American women), and attitudes about AIDS as a genocidal plot (belief that the white power structure deliberately infected blacks with AIDS). Moreover, a national research investigation called "The Violence Initiative: A Gene for Aggression and Young Black Males" (a national conference and U.S. public health initiative, canceled because both would have lend credence to unproved theories on the relationship between genes and violence, thereby legitimating beliefs that black males are genetically prone to violence) help to explain African American mistrust of the medical profession (Dula 1994: 353).

The impact of these cultural historical health care issues can best be seen in a report examining discrimination, race, and health. Williams, Yu, and Jackson

(1997) presented their findings at the 1997 Joint Meeting of the Public Health Conference on Records and Statistics and Data User's Conference in Washington, D.C. Analyzing face-to-face interviews of 1,139 adults residing in Wayne, Oakland, and Macomb Counties in Michigan, these authors revealed that African Americans experienced higher levels of discrimination when compared to European Americans. These experiences of discrimination were generally related to physical and mental health for African Americans, but only to mental health outcomes for European Americans. Williams, Yu, and Jackson state that it has long been known that blacks are exposed to higher levels of discrimination; the research reported here suggests that this burden has important health consequences. Moreover, this report clearly suggests that the time has come for more careful and deliberate investigation of the ways in which social contexts and circumstances, including racial ones, can affect health (Williams, Yu, and Jackson 1997: 22).

CONCLUSION

To critically assess the health status and health issues associated with African Americans, one must use a comprehensive, holistic, biopsychosociocultural approach. This chapter did exactly that—it defined African American culture, provided the most current sociodemographic data; showed how psychosocial issues, religiosity, and health are interrelated and discussed the impact of cultural historical health care issues on African Americans' perception of the health care system. This cultural relativistic perspective to health care is the basic premise of medical anthropology.

POST-EVALUATION QUESTIONS

1. Discuss how African American cultural traits are helpful to African American health outcomes.

2. Describe how cultural issues are connected to each major disease.

3. Discuss the importance of psychosocial and cultural historical issues upon African Americans' perception of the health care system.

REFERENCES

Aschenbrenner, Joyce. 1973. "Extended Families among Black Americans." *Journal of Comparative Family Studies* 4: 257–268.
Baer, Hans. 1985. "Toward a Systematic Typology of Black Folk Healers" *Phylon* 43:327–343.

Bailey, Eric. 1994. "The Health Care Status of African Americans in Indianapo-
    lis." *Journal of the National Medical Association* 86: 853–856.
Berry, Mary and John Blassingame.1982. *Long Memory: The Black Experience
    in America*. New York: Oxford University Press.
Braithwaite, Ronald and Sandra Taylor eds. 1992. *Health Issues in the Black
    Community*. San Francisco: Jossey-Bass.
Chatters, Linda, J. Levin, and C. Ellision. 1998. "Public Health and Health Edu-
    cation in Faith Communities." *Health Education and Behavior* 25:
    689–699.
Dalton, H. 1989. AIDS in Blackface. *Daedalus: Journal of American Academy
    Arts and Science* (Summer): 205–228.
Dula, Annette. 1994. "African American Suspicion of the Healthcare System Is
    Justified: What Do We Do about It?" *Cambridge Quarterly of Health
    Care Ethics* 3: 347–357.
Ellision, Christopher. 1995. "Race, Religious Involvement and Depressive
    Symptomatology in a Southeastern U.S. Community." *Social Science
    and Medicine* 40: 1561–1572.
Franklin, John and Alred Moss. 1988. *From Slavery to Freedom: A History of
    Negro Americans*. New York: Alfred A. Knopf.
Harrison, Ira and Diana Harrion. 1971. "The Black Family Experience and
    Health Behavior." In *Health and the Family: A Medical-Sociological
    Analysis.* Charles O. Crawford, ed. Pp. 175–199. New York: Macmil-
    lan.
Hauser, Joshua. 1997. *Minority Populations and Advance Directives: Insights
    from a Focus Group Methodology.* Pp. 58–74. Cambridge University
    Press.
Jackson, Jacquelyne. 1981. "Urban Black Americans." In *Ethnicity and Medical
    Care*. Alan Harwood, ed. Pp. 37–128. Cambridge. Harvard University
    Press.
Jones, JH. 1981 Bad Blood: *The Tuskegee Syphilis Experiment: A Tragedy of
    Race and Medicine.* New York: Free Press.
Koening H. et al. 1988 *Religion, Health, and Aging.* Westport, CT:
    Greenwood Press.
Levin, Jeffrey. 1996. "How Religion Influences Morbidity and Health: Reflec-
    tions on Natural History, Salutogenesis and Host Resistance." *Social
    Science and Medicine* 43: 849–864.
Levin, Jeffrey, D. Larsen, C. Puchalski. 1997. "Religion and Spirituality in
    Medicine: Research and Education." *Journal of American Medical As-
    sociation* 278: 792–793.
McMiller, William and John Weisz. 1996. "Help-Seeking Preceding Mental
    Health Clinic Intake among African American, Latino, and Caucasian
    Youths." *Journal of American Academy of Child Adolescence Psy-
    chiatry* 35: 8: 1086-1094
McRae, Mary et al.1998. "Black Churches as Therapeutic Systems: A Group
    Process Perspective." *Health Education and Behavior* 25: 778–789.

National Mental Health Association. 1994. "Congressional Briefing Calls Attention to Mental Health Needs of African Americans." *Hospital and Community Psychiatry* 45: 837–838.

Neighbors, Harold. 1991. "Mental Health." In *Life in Black America*. James Jackson, ed. Pp. 221–237. Newbury Park, CA: Sage.

Neighbors, Harold, M. Musick, and D. Williams. 1998. "The African American Minister as a Source of Help for Serious Personal Crises: Bridge or Barrier to Mental Health Care?" *Health Education and Behavior* 25: 759–777.

Picot, Sandra, S. Debanne, K. Namazi, and M. Wykle. 1997. "Religiosity and Perceived Rewards of Black and White Caregivers." *The Gerontologist* 37: 89–101.

Schumaker, J.F. ed. 1992. *Religion and Mental Health*. New York: Oxford University Press.

Stack, Carol. 1974. *All Our Kin: Strategies for Survival in a Black Community*. New York: Harper & Row.

Taylor, R.J. and L. M. Chatters. 1991a. "Non-organizational Religious Participation among Elderly Blacks." *Journal of Gerontology: Social Science*.

———. 1991b. "Religious Life." In *Life in Black America*. James Jackson, ed. Pp. 105–123. Newbury Park, CA: Sage.

Thomas, Stephen and Sandra Quinn. 1991. "The Tuskegee Syphilis Study, 1932 to 1972: Implications for Health Education and AIDS Risk Education Programs in the Black Community." *American Journal of Public Health* 81: 1498–1503.

U.S. Census Bureau. 1996. *Census Bureau Facts for Features*. Washington, DC: U.S. Census Bureau's Public Information Office.

———. 1997. *Census Bureau Facts for Features*. Washington, DC: U.S. Census Bureau's Public Information Office.

———. 1998. *Census Bureau Facts for Features*. Washington, DC: U.S. Census Bureau's Public Information Office.

U.S. Department of Commerce. 1998. *U.S. Census Bureau Facts*. Washington, DC: U.S. Government Printing Office.

Williams, David, Yan Yu and James Jackson. 1997. "Discrimination, Race, and Health." Paper presented at the 1997 Joint Meeting of the Public Health Conference on Records and Statistics and Data User's Conference.

WEB SITES OF SIGNIFICANCE

The Afro-American Newspapers Home Page

http://www.afroam.org

Department of Health & Human Services

http://www.os.dhhs.gov/

Office of Minority Health

http://www.omhrc.gov/

Associate Director for Minority Health

http://www.cdc.gov/od/adhm/

Chapter 4

African American Health Care: A Health Data and Current Research Studies Perspective

CRITICAL THINKING QUESTIONS

1. What are the major diseases associated the African American population?

2. How can African American cultural patterns influence certain disease patterns among African Americans?

3. How can African American cultural patterns improve certain health care outcomes?

INTRODUCTION

This chapter focuses on the major diseases associated with African Americans and the most recent documented research studies investigating African American cultural health issues. According to the National Center for Health Statistics (1997), the ten leading causes of death (from highest incidence to lowest) for African Americans in 1995 were the following:

1. Disease of heart;
2. Malignant neoplasms (cancers);
3. Cerebrovascular diseases (stroke);
4. Human immunodeficiency virus infection (HIV);
5. Unintentional injuries;
6. Homicide and legal intervention;
7. Diabetes mellitus;

8.   Pneumonia and influenza;
9.   Chronic obstructive pulmonary diseases; and
10. Certain conditions originating in the perinatal period. (National Center for
     Health Statistics 1997: 117)

African American men and women, however, differ in the order and rank of the
leading causes of death.

For example, human immunodeficiency virus infection ranked third for
leading causes of death among African American men. With regard to African
American women, cerebrovascular disease and diabetes mellitus ranked third
and fourth, respectively, for leading causes of death. Moreover, ranking ninth
for leading causes of death among African American women were nephritis,
nephrotic syndrome, and nephrosis (lupus). Below are the top ten leading causes
of death for African American men and women (U.S. Department of Health and
Human Services 1997: 118–119).

Black Males: Leading Causes of Death, 1995

All Causes

1.   Diseases of heart
2.   Malignant neoplasms (cancers)
3.   Human immunodeficiency virus infection
4.   Homicide and legal intervention
5.   Unintentional injuries
6.   Cerebrovascular diseases (strokes)
7.   Diabetes mellitus
8.   Pneumonia and influenza
9.   Chronic obstructive pulmonary diseases
10. Certain conditions originating in the perinatal period

Black Females: Leading Causes of Death, 1995

All Causes

1.   Diseases of heart
2.   Malignant neoplasms (cancers)
3.   Cerebrovascular diseases (strokes)
4.   Diabetes mellitus
5.   Human immunodeficiency virus infection
6.   Unintentional injuries
7.   Pneumonia and influenza
8.   Chronic obstructive pulmonary diseases
9.   Nephrities, nephrotic syndrome, and nephrosis (lupus)
10. Certain conditions originating in the perinatal period

In contrast to the U.S. population, the African American population showed a number of different trends in leading causes of death. The following are a few highlights of the 1995 national health statistics:

1. Overall mortality for African Americans continues to be about 60% higher than for European Americans. For most leading causes of death, mortality is higher for African Americans than for other racial and ethnic groups.

2. Compared with European Americans, heart disease mortality was 41% lower for Asian Americans and 49% higher for African Americans in 1995.

3. Between 1990 and 1995, the death rate for cancer declined more for those under 65 years of age than for older persons, more for men than women, and more for black persons than white persons. During this period, among persons 55–64 years of age, cancer mortality declined 12% for black males, 9% for white males, 8% for black females, and 4% for white females.

4. Between 1990 and 1995 breast cancer death rates for black females were relatively stable, following a generally upward trend during the 1980s.

5. Between 1993 and 1995, the homicide rate for young black males 15-24 years of age decreased at an average annual rate of 11% to 132.0 deaths per 100,000 population after increasing at an average annual rate of 12 percent between 1985 and 1992. (National Center for Health Statistics 1997: 6)

To reiterate, the national health statistics data provide a general schematic guideline to assess the past and current trends of the leading causes of death in the U.S. population. Yet when the national health statistics are viewed within a given population, the data can highlight a number of encouraging trends within that population—as depicted in the previous list.

To better understand the major diseases contributing to the death rates associated with African Americans, this next section defines the diseases, highlights an article about the diseases, and shows how cultural factors contribute to those particular diseases. The primary purpose of this discussion is to show the reader that there are always several different ways to approach health data and that any listing of the leading causes of disease must also highlight the cultural factors that most often contribute to such trends.

Heart Disease

Heart disease is the leading cause of death in African men and women. All major causes of heart disease (ischemic, rheumatic, and hypertensive) rise continuously from middle age to old age (*Professional Guide to Diseases* 1998).

Factors that may influence the development of heart disease include cigarette smoking, obesity, physical inactivity, hypertension, diabetes mellitus, and stress (*Professional Guide to Diseases* 1998).

Williams et al. (1997) studied the prevalence of coronary heart disease risk factors among a population of rural African Americans in Virginia and compared their results with current national estimates for African Americans. The study's results found that in their rural African American population, coronary heart disease risk factors were similar to or higher than those reported among African Americans nationally, with the exception of a sedentary lifestyle (817).

The major coronary heart disease risk factors identified were obesity, hypertension, and diabetes. Interestingly, the researchers speculated that cultural perceptions such as the heavier weight is equated with better lifestyle and heavier weight is within African Americans' range of what constitutes healthy contributed to problems of obesity and coronary heart disease.

In another related study, Keil et al. (1995) wanted to determine if racial differences exist in coronary heart disease mortality and coronary risk factors. Data from the two population-based cohorts of the Charleston, South Carolina, and Evans County, Georgia, were pooled to make comparisons of coronary disease mortality and its risk factors. A total of 726 African American men and 1,346 European American men age 35 years or older in 1960 were followed up for 30 years.

Keil et al. (1995) found that the age-adjusted coronary disease mortality was 15% higher among European American men than African American men in Charleston, 50% higher in Evans County, and 30% higher in the combined cohorts. Overall, results from studies in Charleston and Evans County suggest that African American men may experience lower coronary disease mortality than European American men. The risk factors included elevated blood pressure, lower body mass index, lower education, cigarette smoking, and diabetes (1526). Keil et al. (1995) stated that an important contribution of this research has been to identify some of the common risk factors for African Americans and European Americans and that other researchers must unravel the enigma of black-white differences in coronary mortality (1527).

Malignant Neoplasms (Cancer)

Malignant neoplasms (cancer) refer to an abnormal growth of new tissue. The actual cause of neoplasms is not known. Neoplasms may be benign or malignant, depending on their growth pattern. A benign tumor is one that remains circumscribed, although it may vary in size from small to large (*Professional Guide to Diseases* 1998).

A malignant tumor, or cancer, spreads to other cells and tissues and other parts of the body through the bloodstream or lymphatic system. The spreading process is called metastasis. In summary, cancer is a general term for more than 100 diseases, all of which are characterized by the uncontrollable growth of cells (*Professional Guide to Diseases* 1998).

In a national report card for the United States on the cancer incidence and mortality (1973–1995), the American Cancer Society, the National Cancer Institute, and the Centers for Disease Control and Prevention including the National Center for Health Statistics, examined cancer incidence and mortality rates from 1973–1990 and 1990 and 1995 in all racial and ethnic groups in the United States. Wingo et al. (1998) found that for all sites combined, cancer incidence rates decreased on average 0.7% per year during 1990–1995 in contrast to an increasing trend in earlier years. Death rates for the four major cancers (lung, female breast, prostate, and colon/rectum) decreased significantly during 1990–1995 (Wingo et al. 1998:1197).

Examination of incidence rates for each of these sites by race and ethnicity, however, revealed that, except for female breast cancer, African Americans had higher incidence rates than European Americans, Asians and Pacific Islanders, or Hispanics. In particular, breast cancer incidence in African American women continues to increase. Research studies show that breast cancer is diagnosed at later stages in African American women than in European American women, and the five-year relative survival is lower (Miller et al. 1996; Wingo et al. 1998:1205).

With regard to African American men, the incidence of prostate cancer continued to increase. At all ages, African American men tend to be diagnosed with the disease at later stages and to die of prostate cancer more often than European American men do. An estimated 34,400 African American men were diagnosed with prostate cancer in 1996, and 6,400 African American men died from it. The incidence of this disease among African American men is among the highest in the world.

Overall, African American men have an 85% greater risk of developing prostate cancer and a 114% greater risk of dying from the disease than European American men. The reasons for the greater incidence and rate of death among African American men are unknown. However, studies have shown that survival rates among African American men are similar to those among European American men who are treated for the same grade and stage of the disease (American Cancer Society 1998; Polednak 1998; Powell 1994; and Collins 1997).

Interestingly, researchers are gradually examining the relationship of cultural factors to the stage of diagnosis of specific cancers. For example, Lannin et al. (1998) found that cultural factors among African American women influenced their decision to seek care for breast cancer. In a case-control study of patients diagnosed as having breast cancer at the University Medical Center of East Carolina from 1985 through 1992, 540 of 743 patients and 414 control women from the community matched by age, race, and area of residence were interviewed (Lannin et al. 1998:1801).

The cultural factors that seem to be significantly associated with late-stage presentation of breast cancer fell into the following categories: health care utilization, folk beliefs, fundamentalist religious beliefs, relationships with men, perceived risk or fatalism, belief in various treatments for breast cancer, and breast cancer knowledge. Belief that herbs, medicines, or chiropractic are effective treatments for breast cancer also correlated positively with late-stage disease, whereas belief in the effectiveness of surgery was associated with early presentation (Lannin et al. 1998: 1804). Therefore, Lannin et al. contend that the most important effect of the cultural beliefs is that they lead to delayed presentation once a woman has developed a palpable breast abnormality.

Lannin et al. (1998) stated that a significant number of African American women presenting with late-stage disease were reluctant to seek medical treatment for cancer because of their fears about how the disease would impact on their relationships with the men in their lives. These women were afraid that their husbands or male partners would leave them if a cancer diagnosis became known, both because they would no longer be physically attractive but also because they might become burdens to men financially and emotionally (1806).

Finally, Lannin et al. (1998) emphasized that by recognizing that at a least part of the problem is cultural, it may be possible to modify key beliefs in a way that would lead to earlier breast cancer diagnosis and still be consistent with the underlying cultural attributes of the target population (1807).

In the previous study, cultural factors contributed to the poor health outcome of African American women. In the next study, however, cultural factors contribute to the positive health outcome of African American youth. Two studies, in particular, noticed a positive preventive health trend of smoking among African American youths (Flint and Novotny 1998; Robinson and Klesges 1997).

Flint and Novotny (1998) conducted an eleven-year analysis of cigarette smoking among 18–24 year-olds in the United States and found that African Americans became decreasingly at risk to be smokers compared to European Americans. Flint and Novotny speculated that the cause of the differing rates may be that African American adolescents, particularly girls, are less concerned with weight control than are their European American counterparts and therefore less likely to smoke as a form of weight control. Whether this explanation is true or not, Flint and Novotny stated that better understanding of the factors underlying this greater resistance could lead to better smoking prevention strategies for all children and young adults (23).

Robinson and Klesges (1997), on the other hand, highlight specific cultural factors for the differences in smoking onset among African American and European American adolescents. In a comparative study of 6,967 seventh graders in Memphis, Tennessee, Robinson and Klesges found that ethnic difference in smoking prevalence was significant and dramatic: 13% of European Americans were regular smokers versus only 2% of African Americans (501). Additionally, European Americans were 92% more likely than African Americans to view cigarettes as easy to obtain. When controlling for economic factors, this difference still remained between African American and European American adolescents. Thus, given its lower prevalence, Robinson and Klesges showed significant evidence that African American youngsters viewed smoking less favorably.

The results of the Robinson and Klesges study support focus group data from the Office of Minority Health (1997). According to Robert Robinson, CDC's acting associate director for minority health, smoking rates of African American youth have been below those of European Americans, though the rate for young African American males has been increasing. In particular, antismoking sentiment was strongest among African American girls, whose smoking rate has been declining (Office of Minority Health 1997).

The major cultural reasons given by African American girls during the focus groups were that: (1) they felt that they would get in big trouble with their parents for smoking and (2) they disliked the way cigarettes look and smell, and smoking would interfere with their ability to attract boys (Office of Minority Health 1997).

Cerebrovascular Diseases

Cerebrovascular disease, commonly known as stroke, is a sudden impairment of cerebral circulation in one or more of the blood vessels supplying the brain (*Professional Guide to Diseases* 1998). Between 1980 and 1990, stroke had declined rapidly at an average rate of almost 4% per year (National Center for Health Statistics 1997).

According to the National Health Statistics (1994), stroke mortality declined at fairly similar rates for black females, white females, and white males (34% to 36%) and at a slower rate for black males (29%). Yet when age-adjusted death rates are compared, stroke was twice as great for black men as for white men and 80% greater for black women than for white women (NCHS 1994:22).

To investigate the geographic variation in stroke mortality in African Americans and European Americans, Pickle, Mungiole, and Gillum (1997) examined stroke mortality data in the United States from 1988 to 1992. They found considerable geographic variation in stroke mortality for each sex/race group. For instance, they stated that the U.S. age-adjusted stroke death rates per 100,000 for all ages were as follows: black men, 56.6; black women, 43.4; white men, 28.1; white women, 23.8 (1640). Interestingly, patterns of geographic variation coincided with each sex/race group. That is, in African American women and men, high mortality in the southeastern United States persisted. Mortality rates were generally higher in the South than in the North and higher in the East than in the West. Pickle, Mungiole and Gillum stated that compared with data from 1962 to 1988, there was a continuation of the westward shift of high rates to the Mississippi River Valley.

On the other hand, European American women and men showed a spread of areas with high stroke mortality from coastal southeastern states to east south-central and west south central states, including the Mississippi Valley (Pickle, Mungiole, and Gillum 1997: 1641). Compared with the data from 1962 to 1988, Pickle et al. (1997) stated that there was a continuation of the westward shift of high-rate areas to the lower Mississippi River Valley and now westward to Texas. This pattern was more pronounced in European Americans aged 50 than in those aged 70 and 90 years, which suggests that it will continue as the younger cohorts age (Pickle et al. 1997:1641).

Related to the geographic variation of stroke mortality with each sex/race group were the major risk factors that may explain the variation in stroke mortality. Pickle et al. (1997) suggested the following risk factors:

1.   A higher prevalence of hypertension;
2.   A higher prevalence of cigarette smoking;
3.   A diet high in grain-derived complex carbohydrates and sodium; and
4.   A lower access to, and utilization of, preventive health services.

In conclusion, each of these major risk factors most likely contributed to the higher rates of stroke mortality for African Americans and European Americans in each geographic region. Interestingly, Pickle et al's. (1997) findings are supported by Qureshi et al. (1997) and Gillum and Ingram (1996).

In fact, Gillum and Ingram (1996) found that among European Americans, the prevalence of current smoking, abstinence from alcohol, low education, diabetes, history of heart disease, prevalence of hypertension, and residence in a nonmetropolitan area were generally higher in the Southeast than in other regions. Additionally, the prevalence of abstinence from alcohol, low education, residence in a nonmetropolitan area, and mean blood pressure also tended to be higher in the Southeast than in other regions among African Americans. Therefore among both groups (African Americans and European Americans), these risk factors, coupled with a lower access to, and utilization of preventive health services in these areas may contribute to the higher prevalence of stroke in the Southeast (Gillum and Ingram 1996: 671). These findings suggest that efforts directed toward modification of risk factors, particularly hypertension and smoking, could potentially reduce the incidence of stroke and other cerebrovascular diseases (Qureshi et al. 1997).

HIV/AIDS

AIDS, acquired immunodeficiency syndrome, is a disease in which the body's immune system breaks down. The immune system fights off infections and certain other diseases. Because the system fails, a person with AIDS develops a variety of life-threatening illnesses (CDC 1993).

The virus called the human immunodeficiency virus, or HIV, causes AIDS. A virus is a small germ that can cause disease. If HIV enters your bloodstream, you may be infected with HIV. A special blood test can detect HIV infection.

A person who is infected can infect others, even if no symptoms are present. You cannot tell by looking at someone whether he or she is infected with HIV. An infected person can appear completely healthy.

People infected with HIV can develop many health problems. These can include extreme weight loss, severe pneumonia, a form of cancer, and damage to the nervous system. These illnesses signal the onset of AIDS. In some people, these illnesses may develop within a year or two. Others may stay healthy for as long as ten or more years before symptoms appear.

An individual can become infected with HIV in two main ways: (1) having sexual intercourse—vaginal, anal, or perhaps oral with an infected person; and (2) sharing drug needles or syringes with an infected person. Additionally, women infected with HIV can pass the virus to their babies during pregnancy or during birth. In some cases, they can also pass it on when breast-feeding. Blood transfusions infected some people, especially during the period before 1985 when careful screening and laboratory testing of the blood supply began (CDC 1993).

HIV can spread through sexual intercourse, from male to female, female to male, female to female, or male to male. HIV may be in an infected person's blood, semen, or vaginal secretions. It is thought that it can enter the blood-stream through cuts or sores, on tissue in the vagina, penis, or rectum, and possibly through the mouth. Since many infected people have no apparent symptoms of the condition, it's hard to be sure who is or is not infected with HIV. The more sexual partners an individual has, the greater the individual's chances of encountering one who is infected and infecting himself or herself.

African Americans constitute a substantially large percentage of AIDS cases nationally. In 1992, African Americans represented 29% of the reported AIDS cases. In 1993, the AIDS rate for African American females (73 per 100,000) was approximately fifteen times greater than for European American females (5 per 100,00). The rate for African American males in 1993 was five times greater than for European American males. Presently, AIDS is the leading cause of death for African Americans between the ages of 25 and 44 (Centers for Disease Control and Prevention 1994).

In order to examine the attitudes and beliefs associated with HIV/AIDS among African Americans, Nyamathi et al. (1993) investigated the AIDS-related knowledge, perceptions, and behaviors of impoverished African Americans and high-and-low acculturated Latina women. They also attempted to delineate the relationship between knowledge of AIDS, personal characteristics, perceived risk, and risky behaviors among the sampled women (N=1,173) to determine whether risky behaviors differ by race and levels of acculturation.

Nyamathi et al. (1993) found that African American and Hispanic women were equally knowledgeable about AIDS symptomatology; the etiologic agent of AIDS; and behaviors known to reduce risk of HIV infection, such as using condoms and cleaning works used by intravenous drug users. Yet there were major differences between the two groups, with most of the disparity being related to knowledge about modes of transmission.

For instance, African American women and *high-acculturated* (beliefs and behaviors similar to mainstream U.S. society) Hispanics knew that AIDS cannot be acquired from eating foods prepared by a person with AIDS, from being sneezed on by a person with AIDS, or from using toilet seat previously used by a person with AIDS. With respect to the safety of donating blood, African American women were somewhat less knowledgeable than both groups of Hispanic women. In contrast, *low-acculturated* (beliefs and behaviors dissimilar to mainstream U.S. society) Hispanic women were least likely to know of places where one could get tested and were also least likely to be aware that cleaning one's drug paraphernalia with water is not sufficient to kill the AIDS virus.

Overall, the findings of this study indicate that impoverished African American women are very much in need of culturally sensitive counseling about the risks of nonintravenous drug use and sex (especially unprotected) with multiple partners. Nyamathi et al. (1993) stated that the factors that may explain the high prevalence of these risk factors among African American women include early age of sexual intercourse, lack of stable relationships, negative attitudes toward contraception, and greater likelihood of using sex for survival.

Finally, this study provided the first comprehensive data comparing high- and-low acculturated Hispanic and African American women, all of whom are impoverished. It delineated cultural differences in knowledge of AIDS and included information related to perceived risk and actual risk behaviors to provide a basis for planning and evaluating AIDS education programs that truly target specific populations of interest.

In a related study, Thomas and Quinn (1993) examined the attitudes and beliefs about HIV/AIDS among African Americans as it relates to needle exchange programs. A needs assessment of attitudes and beliefs before the implementation of the needle exchange program found the following:

1. Many African Americans are unsure about the degree to which they trust the government reports on AIDS;
2. Many are unsure about the origins of HIV; and
3. Many are unsure or believe that AIDS is a form of genocide against African Americans.

These beliefs help shape the response of many African Americans toward needle exchange programs. Thomas and Quinn (1993) speculated that because of these beliefs as well as other issues, such as the stigmatization of HIV/AIDS, the marginalization of individuals at risk, and the effect of homophobia, it is little wonder that needle exchange programs failed.

Unintentional Injuries

Unintentional injuries consist of fatal accidents at work, home, or recreational sites. Unintentional injury constituted the largest portion of fatal injuries, about 61%, ranging from 50% at ages 20–24 years and 25–34 years to 79–91% for persons 1–9 years of age and 75 years and over. In 1995, 90,402 persons died as a result of unintentional injury, at a crude rate of 34.4 per 100,000 (National Center for Health Statistics 1997:20).

Studies have indicated that African Americans are at high risk of dying from occupational injuries (Loomis and Richardson 1998; Ikeda et al. 1997). Throughout the 1980s, the national rate of occupational fatality was higher for African Americans than for any other group, averaging 6.5 per 100,000 workers, in contrast to 5.8 per 100,000 for European American workers (National

Institute for Occupational Safety and Health 1993; U. S. Department of Health and Human Services 1997; Loomis and Richardson 1998).

To empirically assess whether differences in employment structure and differences in risk within jobs help to explain the racial gap in fatal occupational injury rates, Loomis and Richardson (1998) analyzed African American and European American workers' employment patterns and rates of unintentional fatal injury on the job in North Carolina from 1977 to 1991.

During this period, there were 2,039 unintentional traumatic injuries among eligible African American and European American workers. The number of deaths was largest among European American workers, but the crude injury rate for African Americans was 36% higher after adjustment for age and sex (Loomis and Richardson 1998:41).

Loomis and Richardson (1998) found the following results:

1. African American workers' rate of death from unintentional traumatic injuries on the job was 30% to 50% higher than the rate among European American workers. This differential existed for both men and women.

2. African American men had the highest fatality rate of any group (10.42—Crude rate; European American men—7.90; African American women—0.45; European American women— 0.30).

3. African American women had lower exposure to occupational hazards than European American women.

4. African American women's employment structure leads to higher overall fatality rates.

5. African Americans were somewhat more likely to be employed in several of the most hazardous jobs, including logging, farming, motor transport, and moving services.

6. For men and women combined, the gap in occupational fatality rates would be essentially eliminated if African Americans and European Americans were to work in the same kinds of occupations and industries. (41-42)

In conclusion, the significance of this study to all those who work in high risk occupations can best be summarized in the following statement: "As long as the existence of hazardous jobs is tolerated, the most economically and socially disadvantaged workers will continue to be at the greatest risk" (43).

Homicide

One main source of data on homicides is vital records or death certificates. The information about cause of death on these certificates is assembled and used by local health departments and also is sent to the National Center for Health Statistics to create a national database. The other main source of data on homicides is information collected by police jurisdictions, which assemble these local data and send them to the Federal Bureau of Investigation (FBI). The FBI compiles the data to generate a national profile through the Uniform Crime Reporting Program (Whitman et al. 1996: 782).

In 1995, the homicide rate for young African American males was eight times the rate for young European American males (U.S. Department of Health and Human Services 1997:6; Ikeda et al. 1997). To examine the problem of homicide in the African American population, Whitman et al. (1996) conducted an epidemiological review of homicide data in Chicago. In 1993, there were 850 homicides in Chicago. Whitman et al. (1994) stated that this number corresponds to a crude rate of 31.2 per 100,000 population. The 1992 rate of 34.3 was the highest in the history of Chicago. The epidemiological analysis of the homicide rate, however, revealed some interesting tendencies.

For example, Whitman et al. (1996) found that homicide tends to be perpetrated on members of one's own racial or ethnic group: 93% of homicides committed by non-Hispanic blacks were against non-Hispanic blacks; 74% of homicides committed by non-Hispanic whites were against non-Hispanic whites; and 78% of homicides by Hispanics were committed against Hispanics. Therefore, Whitman et al. suggested that their study contradicted the popular image of homicide. That is, the greatest homicide threats come not from strangers ("stranger danger") but from those we know, even those we love, and from people of the same race and ethnicity.

Finally, Whitman et al. stated that "homicide is connected directly to poverty and disenfranchisement, through their proxy measure of race, and it must be understood that these factors, and many more, cannot be abstracted from the context of the society in which they exist" (785).

Diabetes Mellitus

Diabetes mellitus is a chronic disorder of carbohydrate metabolism resulting from insufficient production of insulin or from inadequate utilization of this hormone by the body's cells (*Professional Guide to Diseases* 1998:849). Diabetes mellitus occurs in four forms classified by etiology: type I (insulin-dependent), type II (noninsulin dependent), other special types (genetic disorder or exposure to certain drugs in chemicals), and gestational diabetes (occurs during pregnancy).

Type I diabetes accounts for 3% of all new cases of diabetes diagnosed each year in the United States. Type I can develop at any age, yet most cases are diagnosed when the individual is under 30 (*Managing Your Diabetes* 1991). Type

II, the more common form of the disease, typically has a gradual onset usually appearing in adults over the age of 40 (*Managing Your Diabetes* 1991). It affects an estimated 85–90% of the 6 million Americans diagnosed with diabetes. The likelihood of developing type II is approximately equal by sex but is greater in African Americans, Hispanics, and Native Americans. Major risk factors include a family history of diabetes, obesity, age 40 or over, hypertension, gestational diabetes, or having one or more infants weighing more than nine pounds at birth (*Professional Guide to Diseases* 1998).

Diabetes mellitus is a major clinical and public health problem in the African American community. African American men have a prevalence of diabetes that is 80% higher than that for European American men, while African American women have a prevalence 90% higher than that for European American women (Herman et al. 1998: 147) In addition, in 1990, age adjusted rate of hospitalization related to diabetes for African American women was 22% higher than for African American men, 215% higher than for European American women, and 213% higher than for European American men (Herman et al. 1998:148.). These diabetes statistics indicate that not only are there distinctive differences between African Americans and European Americans in the prevalence and hospitalization rates associated with diabetes but also research is needed to determine if any other factors, such as social and cultural that may be contributing to the large disparity of diabetes-related problems.

In a study to determine differences in self-reported adherence to a dietary regimen, Fitzgerald et al. (1997) surveyed 178 African American and European American patients at a Michigan suburban endocrinology clinic from 1993 to 1994. They found that the two groups of patients with noninsulin dependent diabetes (NIDDM) reported similar adherence to dietary recommendations; similar overall adherence, beliefs, and attitudes as measured by their diabetes care profile scale; and a similar percent ideal body weight (Fitzgerald et al. 1997: 46).

Further analyses, however, revealed that African Americans and European Americans differed in the perception of diabetes and the perception of dietary adherence to the dietary regimen to diabetes. Fitzgerald et al. (1997) speculated that among African American women the motivation to lose weight often is not for health reasons but for improved appearance. The importance of weight loss to one's diabetic condition is de-emphasized, and more value is placed upon losing weight for improved appearance. If weight loss does not occur, then negative beliefs and attitudes may decrease the individual's motivation and promote a "why bother" attitude thereby leading to nonadherence to the dietary regimen for diabetes (Fitzgerald et al. 1997: 46).

To counteract this "why bother" attitude as it relates to weight loss and dietary adherence, Fitzgerald et al. (1997) suggested that health educators need to help patients recognize their feelings about diabetes, identify the ways that their feelings influence their behaviors, and develop strategies for coping with their feelings. The cultural/social functions of food and what food "means" and "symbolizes" to the individual should be considered when developing meal plans and educational interventions for the African American diabetic patient.

In order to examine more of the underlying cultural health beliefs associated with diabetes mellitus, Maillet et al. (1996) conducted a focus group of African American women with noninsulin dependent diabetes mellitus (NIDDM) and those at risk for noninsulin dependent diabetes mellitus. Six African American women with noninsulin dependent diabetes mellitus and one African American woman at risk for noninsulin dependent diabetes mellitus participated in the focus group meetings. The focus group was conducted within the district of a northeastern urban medical university in a relaxed and informal classroom (40).

The major themes that emerged from the focus groups were the importance of family and social support, a propensity to binge or overeat when food restrictions were placed by family members, difficulties with dietary changes, inability to develop an exercise regimen because of multiple barriers, lack of clarity about diabetes complications, prevention of complications valued but not widely understood, and a need for future programs that are culturally sensitive to African American women (Maillet et al. 1996: 44). Furthermore, a consistent theme of this focus group was that family support or a lack of support had an impact on one's stated ability to make dietary modifications (45).

Specifically, Maillet et al. suggested that older African American women find it difficult to make dietary changes because changing their diet disrupts a lifetime of culture within the context of family. Culture may directly influence diabetes education and must be understood and incorporated into intervention programs to encourage success (Maillet et al. 1996: 45). Therefore, when providing care to African American women (young, middle-age, and mature), Maillet et al. (1996) suggested that the primary health care providers must be sensitive to the role that culture plays in diet, weight loss, and diabetes self-management.

Finally, the former President of the National Medical Association, Yvonnecris Smith Veal (1996) states that there are three basic reasons why diabetes continues to plague the African American community. First, there are the lifestyle and behavioral patterns associated with African Americans, such as poor eating habits, obesity, limited access to adequate medical care, and limited funds. African Americans in general tend to eat foods high in calories and loaded with saturated fats and sugar, along with having a sedentary lifestyle— all of which are contributing factors to being overweight. Second, African Americans have a history of preparing foods with lard and other heavy oils. This type of food preparation, along with the inability to obtain a balanced diet, contributes to the risk factors associated with diabetes. Third, African Americans need more options to choose dietary diabetic regimens that fit the preferences for certain foods and eating practices among all segments of the African American population (203).

Pneumonia and Influenza

Pneumonia is defined as an acute infection of the alveolar spaces or inter-stitial tissues (or both) of the lung (*Professional Guide to Diseases* 1998). There are four classifications of pneumonia: typical, or classical bacteria pneumonia; atypical pneumonia; aspiration pneumonia; and hematogenous pneumonia.

Microorganisms such as bacteria and viruses may cause pneumonia. Most pneumonias in children are viral and require symptomatic treatment. Pneumonia in adults presents in two general ways, as "typical" pneumonia and as "atypical" pneumonia. Atypical pneumonias are milder and slower in onset, whereas typi-cal pneumonias are more severe and abrupt in onset *(Professional Guide to Dis-eases* 1998).

Pneumonia is the sixth leading cause of death among European Americans and the eighth leading cause among African Americans (NCHS 1997: 117). African American men, however, had a higher (58%) pneumonia mortality rate compared to European American men; the corresponding figure for African American women was 26% higher than for European American women (Na-tional Heart, Lung, and Blood Institute 1995: 1386).

To examine the disparity of pneumonia-related deaths between African Americans and European Americans, Marston et al. (1997) investigated the in-cidence of community-acquired pneumonia of all adults from two counties in Ohio who were hospitalized in 1991. Based on a sample of 2,776 patients who met the study's criteria, Marston et al. found the following results:

1. Pneumonia incidence was higher among blacks than white (337.7/100,000 vs. 253.9/100,000);

2. Pneumonia incidence in persons younger than 45 years was more than twice for blacks compared to whites;

3. Pneumonia incidence in persons 65 years or older was similar for blacks and whites;

4. Pneumonia incidence was higher among men (291.4/100,00) than women (244.8/100,000); and

5. Deaths from pneumonia were similar among blacks (8.2%) and whites (8.9%). (1712)

Interestingly, Marston et al. speculated that the dramatic differences in the rates of pneumonia in certain populations may, in part, be due to differences in socio-economic status. In conclusion, their findings should prompt investigation of the bases for racial differences in pneumonia rates and may warrant reconsideration of recommendations for the use of pneumococcal vaccination and other preven-tion strategies (1715).

Chronic Obstructive Pulmonary Disease

The term "chronic obstructive pulmonary disease" is applied to the condition of permanent airflow obstruction associated with significant physiologic impairment (NHLBI 1995: 1384). Diseases that may lead to chronic obstructive pulmonary disease include emphysema, chronic bronchitis, chronic asthma, bronchiectasis, silicosis, and pulmonary tuberculosis (*Professional Guide to Diseases* 1998: 534).

In 1995, the age-adjusted death rate for chronic obstructive pulmonary diseases was 54% higher for males than females (26.3 and 17.1 deaths per 100,000, respectively). The chronic obstructive pulmonary disease death rates were highest for the elderly and have been increasing most rapidly among females age 75 years and over (NCHS 1997:6).

In 1995, while chronic obstructive pulmonary disease was the fourth leading cause of death among all Americans, it was only the ninth leading cause of death among African Americans (NCHS 1997:117). The National Heart, and Lung Blood Institute (NHLBI) Working Group (1995) stated that since the prevalence for chronic obstructive pulmonary disease has been lower for African Americans, there have been only a small number of studies investigating this health care issue. In fact, the NHLBI Working Group emphasized that future studies on minority populations need to elucidate how the effects of genetic, environmental, and socioeconomic factors relate to the prevalence of chronic obstructive pulmonary disease (NHLBI 1995: 1384).

As stated earlier, chronic asthma is a disease that may lead to chronic obstructive pulmonary disease. About 13 million people in the United States are estimated to have asthma (NHLBI 1995). Asthma prevalence among adults has increased steadily since 1982 in all age groups. Similarly, the prevalence of asthma in adult African Americans has increased from 39/1,000 in 1982 to 53/1,000 persons in 1989 (NHLBI 1995:1382).

The NHLBI report (1995) stated that asthma is also increasing in African American children. The prevalence of asthma among 6-to 11-year-old African American children was 9.4%, compared with 6.2% in European American children (1382). Moreover, the asthma mortality rates are four to seven times higher for young African Americans (age 5 to 34 years) than for young European Americans.

To examine the cultural factors that may be related to the higher prevalence and mortality rate of asthma among African American children, Dinkevich et al. (1998) investigated parents' perceptions of asthma in an inner-city hospital emergency department. The results of this self-administered, 30-item questionnaire given to 466 parents of patients less than eighteen years of age attending the pediatric emergency department of Jacobi Medical Center, a municipal hospital in Bronx, New York, were as follows:

1. Over 90% of respondents reported a source of primary medical care for their child;

2. Eighty-nine percent of parents whose children received their usual asthma care from their primary care provider reported that they could get an appointment with their child's regular doctor on the same day compared with 67.3% of parents whose children got most of their asthma care from the emergency department;

3. Only 33% of parents attempted to call or go to their child's doctor's office prior to the current emergency department visit; and

4. Fifty percent came directly to the emergency department. (Dinkevich et al. 1998: 67)

Dinkevich et al. (1998) suggested that the reasons so few African American parents chose to contact their child's regular doctor prior to the emergency department visit may be related to the perceived severity of the asthma attack at the time of presentation, the lack of parental confidence in the efficacy of asthma medications, the availability and perceived quality of emergency department care, and limited understanding of asthma management (67). Furthermore, since nearly all inner-city children with asthma using the emergency department can identify a regular health care provider, Dinkevich et al. recommended that efforts to improve the delivery of effective asthma care in the primary care settings may contribute to reducing asthma morbidity and excessive emergency department use.

In another related study on the perceptions of asthma, Luder et al. (1998) examined the association of being overweight with greater asthma symptoms in inner-city African American and Hispanic children in New York City's East Harlem and South Bronx neighborhoods. They found that their sample of children with asthma had a higher prevalence of overweight compared with their peers from the same environment. Luder et al. also found that asthma severity in the study subjects contributed to overweight because of imposed limitations on physical activity.

Luder et al. speculated that most parents believed that a child with asthma should never exercise. In fact, children with asthma can and should exercise in accordance with their height, weight, and age. Thus, parents' perceptions of asthma management and being overweight may have influenced the increased prevalence of asthma attacks among this sample of African American and Hispanic American children.

Certain Conditions Originating in the Perinatal Period

Certain conditions originating in the perinatal period refer to deaths associated with childbirth. Perinatal loss involves perinatal mortality, both stillbirth and neonatal death.

In 1995, the infant mortality rate was 7.6 deaths per 1,000 live births, a record low. During the period 1990 through 1995, the infant mortality rate for black infants was 2.4 times the rate for white infants (U.S. Department of health and Human Services 1997:5). Although the black infant mortality rate has stabilized in recent years, the disparity between black and white infant mortality remains a perplexing multifactorial health care problem.

For example, Zambrana and Scrimshaw (1997) investigated the associations between psychosocial factors and patterns of substance use within ethnic groups and assessed maternal sociodemographic, prenatal, and psychosocial factors of women who continue to use substances during pregnancy and those who do not. Face-to-face interviews were conducted with African American (N=255), Mexican American (N=525), and Mexican immigrant (N=764) women in 22 community-based prenatal care clinics in Los Angeles County during the years 1987-1990 (254).

Zambrana and Scrimshaw found significant ethnic differences in the use of alcohol, cigarettes, and illicit drugs. Their sample of low-income women with a mean educational level of 11.52 years (African Americans), 10.46 years (Mexican Americans) and 8.18 years (Mexican immigrants) exhibited the following social and cultural characteristics:

1. African American women reported more stressful life events, more distress from these events, and higher anxiety than Mexican-origin respondents.

2. Mexican-origin respondents were more likely to report money worries, a change in residence, and robberies or burglaries than were African American women.

3. African American and Mexican American women were more likely than Mexican immigrants to report support from the family. (256)

These social and cultural characteristics appear to have influenced the substance use behavior of the sampled women. Zambrana and Scrimshaw found that African American women were more likely (25%) than Mexican-origin women (7.6%) to report use of substances before and during pregnancy. Mexican American women were more likely than Mexican immigrant women to report use of substances before and during pregnancy. Finally, African American women were twice as likely (10.6%) as Mexican American women (5.0%) to report use of all three substances (alcohol, drugs, cigarettes), while less than 1% of the Mexican immigrant respondents reported use of all three substances (257).

The impact of this study to prenatal care and African American deaths originating in the perinatal period can be best summarized as follows:

There is a need to explore, among African American women, the nature of socio-environmental factors that are contributing to such high levels of psychosocial stress. We need to focus inquiry on those institutional, community, and family-related intervening or mediating factors within ethnic groups that promote positive health behaviors and decrease risk for substance use (Zambrana and Scrimshaw 1997).

Nephritis, Nephrotic Syndrome and Nephrosis: (ex. Lupus)

Lupus is defined as a chronic inflammatory disorder of the connective tissue (erythematosus) that appears in two forms: one that affects only the skin, and another that affects multiple organ systems, as well as the skin (*Professional Guide to Diseases* 1998: 366). Recurring remissions and exacerbations, especially common during the spring and summer, characterize systemic lupus erythematosus (SLE).

The annual incidence of lupus (SLE) averages 75.4 cases per 1 million African Americans and 27.5 cases per 1 million European Americans. Lupus is also eight times more common among women and fifteen times more common during childbearing years (*Professional Guide to Diseases* 1998: 366).

The exact cause of lupus is unknown, yet current evidence suggests that multiple factors such as hormones, genetics, immunology, and environment are the major causative agents. For African Americans, lupus has become a major health care and mortality issue that needs prompt attention by clinicians and health care researchers.

For example, McCarty et al. (1995) examined racial differences in the incidence of systemic lupus erythematosus (SLE) residents of Allegheny County, Pennsylvania, which includes the Pittsburgh metropolitan area. The study period ranged from January 1, 1985, to December 31, 1990. Only lupus patients who were living in Allegheny County at least six months prior to diagnosis were accepted for inclusion in their study.

McCarty et al. (1995) identified 191 incident cases of definite lupus diagnosed in this period. Examining differences by sex revealed that the incidence of definite SLE was 9 times higher in white females compared with white males and 13 times higher in African American females compared with African American males (1263). When examined by race, the incidence in African American females was 2.5 times higher than that in white females. In males, the incidence in African Americans was almost twice as high as that in whites.

To account for the different incidence rates, McCarty et al. could not identify specific causative elements. However, they did suggest that future studies are necessary to determine whether these differences may be due, in part, to socioeconomic factors or issues related to care and whether African American patients with SLE are being seen by primary care physicians but not being referred to a specialist (1268). The next study accomplished this very task.

Kardestuncer and Frumkin (1997) conducted a field investigation of lupus in an African American community in Gainsville, Georgia. Interestingly, a community group, the Newton Florist Club, initiated this study, because members suspected that the community had an increased prevalence of lupus (85).

Interviewers collected data through a community survey, which was administered to one reliable adult respondent in each participating home. The survey contained information about demographics for each household resident, dates of residence, and medical information (86).

Kardestuncer and Frumkin surveyed a total of 81 households and collected information about 246 current and past inhabitants. They found 4 cases of lupus: 3 in current residents and 1 in a former resident who had moved in 1990 and had been diagnosed in 1994. Compared with the U.S. population incidence rates (1.8 to 4.6 cases/100,000 persons), the Newton community had a ninefold increase in incidence (p=.0001).

Although this study had several shortcomings (sample size, inability to track potential cases, no control over community), Kardestuncer and Frumkin emphasized that their findings support the hypothesis that environmental toxins may induce lupus. The fact that this study population was located in the industrial southern part of the town where several plants resided, including a scrap iron and metal company, a soybean mill and oil refinery, a feed mill, a wood pressure treatment plant, a wood-products facility, and a tank and equipment company, provided support for their hypothesis. In addition, in the 1930s, Newton was built atop a former city landfill in which municipal and industrial waste may have been deposited. With such supportive cultural historical data, Kardestuncer and Frumkin contended that the incidence rates of lupus among African Americans in Newton are directly related to the environmental toxins located in this community.

In conclusion, Kardestuncer and Frumkin suggested that local health care providers should become thoroughly familiar with environmental issues, including basic environmental toxicology, the community's exposure profile, symptoms of important environmental syndromes, and information resources. Additionally, medical screening for the detection of both evidence of exposures and evidence of early disease should be considered; such initiative should be designed on the basis of the community's past exposures and current disease profile (88).

Sickle-Cell Anemia

Sickle-cell anemia results from a defective hemoglobin molecule that causes red blood cells (RBCs) to roughen and become sickle-shaped (*Professional Guide to Diseases* 1998). Sickle-cell disease is a generic term for a group of genetic disorders characterized by the predominance of hemoglobin S. Sickle-cell disorders include sickle-cell anemia and the sickle-B thalassemia syndromes in which hemoglobin S is associated with another abnormal hemoglobin (NHLBI 1995: 1387).

Sickle-cell disorders are found in people of African, Mediterranean, Native American, and Middle Eastern heritages. The incidence rate for African Americans is 1:540 births (1,189 cases each year), in whom sickle-cell anemia and its variants are a substantial cause of major illness. Additionally, the frequency of the sickle-cell trait varies from 8% to 12% of the population, whereas overt sickle-cell anemia affects 1 in every 300 to 400 African Americans (NHLBI 1995).

To examine the national trend in the mortality of children with sickle-cell disease from 1968 through 1992, Davis et al. (1997) reviewed death certificate data obtained from the Cooperative Study of Sickle Cell Disease. Information on deaths of one-to fourteen-year-old African American children with sickle-cell disease for the period 1968 through 1992 was extracted from computer tapes containing death certificate data on all deaths in the United States.

Davis et al. found that among children in each annual birth cohort (each year from 1969 to 1985), an estimated average of 55 died when they were one to four years old, a mortality rate of 37 deaths per 1,000 African American children with sickle cell disease. By the time African American children with sickle-cell disease born 1986 through 1988 were one to four years old, each annual birth cohort had an average of 36 deaths in this age group, and the mortality rate had decreased 41% to 22 deaths per 1,000 children with sickle-cell disease in the cohort (1319). Therefore, the Davis et al. study demonstrated marked decreases in rates of death of African American children with sickle- cell disease, with decreasing trends shown in all childhood age groups.

Interestingly, the major cause for the declining deaths associated with sickle-cell disease is the result of the 1972 National Sickle Cell Anemia Control Act, which established a sickle cell disease research program organized and sponsored by the National Institutes of Health (Davis et al. 1997: 1321). Davis et al. (1997) stated that research conducted under this program resulted in a better understanding and awareness of how to prevent deaths of children with sickle cell disease and how to develop new educational outreach programs for local African American populations throughout the United States.

Alzheimer's Disease

Alzheimer's disease, also called primary degenerative dementia, is a deterioration of mental capacity. Alzheimer's disease accounts for over half of all dementias. Causative factors of Alzheimer's disease include neurochemical, environmental (aluminum and manganese), viral (slowly growing central nervous system virus), trauma, and genetic immunology (*Professional Guide to Diseases* 1998: 638).

The overall age-adjusted death rate from Alzheimer's disease increased to 2.3 deaths per 100,000 in 1993. Rates increased rapidly from 1979 to 1988 before leveling off between 1988 and 1992 (NCHS 1996).

Death rates from Alzheimer's disease increase with age. For Americans aged 65–74 years, the death rate was nearly 10 deaths per 100,000 population. For persons aged 75–84 years, the rate increased to 64 per 100,000 population, and for those age 85 years and over it was almost 228 per 100,000 population (NCHS 1996).

Age-adjusted death rates from Alzheimer's disease were greater for males than for females, but the differences in rates by sex decreased substantially from

1979 to 1993. Age-adjusted rates were nearly two times higher for the European American population than for the African American population (NCHS 1996).

To determine the medical, social, and cultural pattern of Alzheimer's disease among African Americans, Gorelick (1994) studied 113 African American Alzheimer's disease (AD) patients and 79 African American vascular dementia (VaD) patients in Chicago. They found that the typical demographic and background profile of their African American AD and VaD patients was that of a woman born in the southern portion of the United States who had lived on a farm until her mid-teenage years before moving to Chicago. These women currently lived in a house or apartment with other family members, were retired, widowed, and Protestant, and had some form of medical insurance. Furthermore, the mean number of years of education was 9.1 for AD patients and 9.4 for VaD patients. AD patients were generally older than VaD patients (76.4 vs 71.8 years, p = 0.0109) and remained in their state of birth for a greater length of time before moving to Chicago than VaD patients (26.3 versus 18.8 years, p = 0.0263) (1393).

In summary, this study represents one of the few research initiatives that exclusively target African American patients with AD and VaD. In fact, the Gorelick study provided one of the best comprehensive and detailed epidemiological analyses of baseline frequency and comparison of risk factors among African Americans with these two important diseases. Since the older adult segment of the African American population will continue to increase, more comprehensive and culturally sensitive studies of Alzheimer's disease among African Americans is warranted.

In fact, increasing patient diversity in studies of Alzheimer's disease is needed if clinicians are to fully understand the full clinical manifestations of the disease and its social consequences in all segments of our society (Welsh et al. 1994: 46). Welsh et al. (1994) contended that this very basic information is needed for advancing clinicians' and health care researchers' understanding of the pathogenesis of the disease, estimating disease prevalence, and accurately gauging future health care costs and needs across all sectors of the population.

CONCLUSION

In summary, in order to critically assess the health status and disease patterns of African Americans, one must use a comprehensive, holistic, biopsychosociocultural approach. The holistic approach to health care is the basic premise of medical anthropology. This chapter concentrates upon the major causes of death and the cultural issues associated with each disease.

POST-EVALUATION QUESTIONS

1. Discuss the major leading causes of death among African American men and women.

2. Discuss the type of cultural patterns among African American men and women that may contribute to their disease patterns.

3. Why is it important to determine the interrelationship between cultural practices with disease patterns among African Americans?

REFERENCES

American Cancer Society. 1998. *Cancer Facts and Figures–1998*. Atlanta: American Cancer Society.

Bailey, Eric. 1991. *Urban African American Health Care*. Lanham, MD: University Press of America.

Baker, F.M. 1982. "Ethnic and Cultural Variations in the Care of the Aged. Discussion: The Black Elderly: Biopsychosocial Perspective Within an Age Cohort and Adult Development Context." *Journal of Geriatric Psychiatry* 15: 225–237.

Bennett, Charles et al. 1995. "Racial Differences in Care among Hospitalized Patients with Pneumocystis Carinii Pneumonia in Chicago, New York, Los Angeles, Miami, and Raleigh-Durham." *Archives Internal Medicine* 155: 1586–1592.

Berry, Mary and John Blassingame.1982. *Long Memory: The Black Experience in America*. New York: Oxford University Press.

Braithwaite, Ronald and Sandra Taylors. eds. 1992. *Health Issues in the Black Community*. San Francisco: Jossey-Bass.

Centers for Disease Control and Prevention. 1993a. *Facts about HIV/AIDS and Race/Ethnicity*. Washington, DC: U.S. Government Printing Office.

———. 1993b. *AIDS Prevention Guide*. Washington, DC: U.S. Government Printing Office.

Chatters, Linda, J. Levin, and C. Ellison. 1998. "Public Health and Health Education in Faith Communities." *Health Education & Behavior* 25: 689–699.

Collins, M. 1997. "Increasing Prostate Cancer Awareness in African American Men." *Oncology Nursing Forum* Jan/Feb. 24: 91–95.

Dalton, H.S. 1998. "AIDS in Blackface." *Daedalus* 1989: 118: 220.

Davis, Harold, K. Schoendorf, P. Gergen, and R. Moore. 1997. "National Trends in the Mortality of Children with Sickle Cell Disease, 1968 through 1992." *American Journal of Public Health* 87: 1317–1322.

Dinkevich, Eugene, S. Cunningham, and E. Crain. 1998. "Parental Perceptions of Access to Care and Quality of Care for Inner-City Children with Asthma." *Journal of Asthma* 35: 63–71.

Dula, Annette. 1994. "African American Suspicion of the Healthcare System Is Justified: What Do We Do about It?" *Cambridge Quarterly of Healthcare Ethics* 3: 347–357.

Ellison, Christopher. 1995. "Race, Religious Involvement and Depressive Symptomatology in a Southeastern U.S. Community." *Social Science and Medicine* 40: 1561–1572.

Fitzgerald, James, R. Anderson, M Funnell, M. Arnold, W. Davis, L. Aman, S. Jacober, and Grunberger. 1997. "Differences in the Impact of Dietary Restrictions on African Americans and Caucasians with NIDDM." *The Diabetes Educator* 23: 41–47.

Flint, Alan and Thomas Novotny. 1998. "Trends in Black/White Differences in Current Smoking among 18- to 24 Year-Olds in the United States, 1983–1993." *American Journal of Preventive Medicine* 14: 19-24.

Franklin, John and Alfred Moss. 1988. *From Slavery to Freedom: A History of Negro Americans.* New York: Alfred A. Knopf.

Gillum, Richard and Deborah Ingram. 1996. "Relation between Residence in the Southwest Region of the United States and Stroke Incidence: The NHANES I Epidemiological Analyses." *American Journal of Epidemiology* 144: 665-673.

Gilthorpe, M.S. 1998. "Variations in Hospitalization Rates for Asthma among Blacks and Minority Ethnic Communication." *Respiratory Medicine* 92: 642–648.

Gorelick, P.B., S. Freels, B.A. Harris, T. Dollear, M. Billingsley, and N. Brown. 1994. "Epidemiology of Vascular and Alzheimer's Dementia among African Americans in Chicago, IL." *Neurology* 44: 1391–1396.

Harrison, Ira and Diana Harrison. 1971. "The Black Family Experience and Health Behavior." In *Health and the Family: A Medical-Sociological Analysis,* Charles O. Crawford. New York: Macmillan.

Hauser, Joshua. 1997. "Minority Populations and Advance Directives: Insights from a Focus Group Methodology." *Cambridge Quarterly of Health Care Ethics* 6: 58–74

Herman, William, T. Thompson, W. Visscher, R. Aubert, M. Engelgau, L. Liburd, D. Watson, and T. Hartwell. 1998. "Diabetes Mellitus and Its Complement in an African American Community: Project DIRECT." *Journal of National Medical Association* 90: 147–156.

Ikeda, Robin, R. Gorwitz, S. James, K. Powell, and J. Mercy. 1997. "Trends in Fatal Firearm-Related Injuries, United States, 1962–1993." *American Journal of Preventive Medicine* 13: 396–400.

Jackson, Jacquelyne. 1981. "Urban Black Americans." In *Ethnicity and Medical Care.* Alan Harwood, ed. Pp. 37–128 Cambridge: Harvard University Press..

Jones, JH. 1981. *Bad Blood: The Tuskegee Syphilis Experiment: A Tragedy of Race and Medicine.* New York: Free Press.

Kardestuncer, Tarik and Howard Frumkin. 1997. "Systemic Lupus Erythematosus in Relation to Environmental Pollution: An Investigation in an African American Community in North Georgia." *Archives of Environmental Health* 52: 85–90.

Keil, Julian, S. Sutherland, C. Hames, D. Lackland, P. Gazes, R. Knapp, and H.
Tyroler. 1995. "Coronary Disease Mortality and Risk Factors in Black
and White Men." *Archives of Internal Medicine* 155: 1521–1527.

Koening H., M. Smiley, and J. Gonzales. 1988. *Religion, Health, and Aging.*
Westport, CT: Greenwood Press.

Lannin D. R., H. Mathews, J. Mitchell, M. Swanson, F. Swanson, and E. Edwards. 1998. "Influence of Socioeconomic and Cultural Factors on Racial Differences in Late-Stage Presentation of Breast Cancer." *Journal
of American Medical Association* 279: 1801–1807.

Levin, Jeffrey. 1996. "How Religion Influences Morbidity and Health: Reflections on Natural History, Salutogenesis and Host Resistance." *Social
Science and Medicine* 43: 849-864.

Levin, J., D. Larson, and C. Puchalski. 1997. "Religion and Spirituality in
Medicine: Research and Education." *Journal of American Medical Association* 278: 792–793

Loomis, Dana and David Richardson. 1998. "Race and the Risk of Fatal Injury
at Work." *American Journal of Public Health* 88: 40–44.

Luder, Elisabeth et al. 1998. "Association of Being Overweight with Greater
Asthma Symptoms in Inner City Black and Hispanic Children." *The
Journal of Pediatrics* 132: 699–703.

Maillet, Nancy, G. Melkus, and G. Spollett. 1996. "Using Focus Groups to
Characterize the Health Beliefs and Practices of Black Women with
Non-Insulin Dependent Diabetes." *The Diabetes Educator* 22: 39–46.

Managing Your Diabetes. 1991. Indianapolis, IN: Eli Lilly and Company.

Marston, Barbara et al. 1997. "Incidence of Community-Acquired Pneumonia
Requiring Hospitalization." *Archives of Internal Medicine* 157: 1709–
1718.

McCarty, Daniel, S. Manzi, T. Medsger, R. Ramsey-Goldman, R. LaPorte, and
C. Kwoh. 1995. "Incidence of Systemic Lupus Erythematosus: Race
and Gender Differences." *Arthritis and Rheumatism* 38: 1260–1270.

McKenna, Matthew et al. 1998. "The Fall after the Rise: Tuberculosis in the
United States, 1991 through 1994." *The American Public Health Association* 88:1059–1063.

McMiller, William and John Weisz. 1996. "Help-Seeking Preceding Mental
Health Clinic Intake among African American, Latino, and Caucasian
Youths." *Journal of American Academy of Child Adolescence Psy-
chiatry* 35: 1086–1094.

McRae, Mary et al. 1998. "Black Churches as Therapeutic Systems: A Group
Process Perspective." *Health Education & Behavior* 25: 778–789.

Miller B., L. Kolonel, L. Berstein, L. Young, G. Swanson, D. West, C. Key, J. Liff, C. Glover, G. Alexander et al. (eds.) 1996. *Racial/Ethnic Patterns of Cancer in the United States 1988–1992*. Bethesda, MD: National Cancer Institute; NIH publication 96-4104.

National Center for Health Statistics. 1996. "Mortality Trends for Alzheimer's Disease: Fact Sheets." *Vital and Health Statistics*, Series 20, No. 28. Centers for Disease Control and Prevention.

National Center for Health Statistics. 1997. *Health United States 1996-97 and Injury Chartbook*. Hyattsville, MD: DHHS publication PHS 97-1232.

National Heart, Lung and Blood Institute. 1995. "Respiratory Diseases Disproportionately Affecting Minorities." *Chest* 108: 1380–1392.

National Institute for Occupational Safety and Health. 1993. *Fatal Injuries to Workers in the United States, 1980-1989: A Decade of Surveillance, National and State Profiles*. Cincinnati, OH: DHHS publication NIOSH 93-108S.

National Mental Health Association. 1994. "Congressional Briefing Calls Attention to Mental Health Needs of African Americans." *Hospital and Community Psychiatry* 45: 837–838.

Nyamathi, A., C. Bennett, B. Leake, C. Lewis, and J. Flaserud. 1993. "AIDS-Related Knowledge, Perceptions and Behaviors among Impoverished Minority Women." *American Journal of Public Health* 12: 339-346.

Office of Minority Health Resource Center. 1997. "African Americans Girls Less Interested in Smoking." News from Sessions at the Sixth Biennial Symposium on Minorities, the Medically Underserved, and Cancer, April 23–27, U.S. Department of Health and Human Services.

Parker, Vanessa, S. Sussman, D. Crippen, D. Scholl, and P. Elder. 1996. "Qualitative Development of Smoking Prevention Programming for Minority Youth." *Addictive Behaviors* 21: 521–525.

Pickle, Linda, M. Mungiole, and R. Gillum. 1997. "Geographic Variation in Stroke Mortality in Blacks and Whites in the United States." *Stroke* 28: 1639–1647.

Picot, Sandra, S. Debanne, K. Namazi, and M. Wykle. 1997. "Religiosity and Perceived Rewards of Black and White Caregivers." *The Gerontologist* 37: 89–101.

Polednak, A.P. 1998. "Prostate Cancer Treatment in Black and White Men: The Need to Consider Both Stage at Diagnosis and Socioeconomic Status." *Journal of the National Medical Association* 90: 101–104.

Powell, IJ. 1994. "Early Detection Issues of Prostate Cancer in African American Men." *In Vivo* 8: 451–452.

Professional Guide to Diseases. 1998 Springhouse, PA: Springhouse.

Qureshi, Adnan, M. Suri, K. Safdar, J. Ottenlips, R. Janssen, and M. Frankel. 1997. "Intracerebral Hemorrhage in Blacks." *Stroke* 28: 961–964.

Robinson, Leslie and Robert Klesges. 1997. "Ethnic and Gender Differences in Risk Factors for Smoking Onset." *Health Psychology* 16: 499–505.

Schumaker, J.F. ed. 1992 *Religion and Mental Health*. New York: Oxford University Press.

Thomas, Stephen and Sandra Quinn. 1991. "The Tuskegge Syphilis Study, 1932 to 1972: Implications for Health Education and AIDS Risk Education Programs in the Black Community." *American Journal Public Health* 81: 1498–1503.

———. 1993. "An Evaluation of HIV Education Messengers in a Black Low-Income Housing Complex. " *Journal of Health Education* 24: 135–140.

U.S. Department of Commerce. 1998. *U.S. Census Bureau Facts.* Washington, DC: U.S. Government Printing Office.

U.S. Department of Health & Human Services. 1997. *Health. United States 1996-97 and Injury Chartbook.* National Center for Health Statistics. Washington, DC: U.S. Government Printing Office. DHHS Publication No.:97-1232.

Veal, Yvonnecris. 1996. "African Americans and Diabetes: Reasons, Rationale, and Research." *Journal of the National Medical Association* 88: 203–204.

Welsh, K.A, E. Ballard, F. Nash, K. Raiford, and L. Harrell. 1994. "Issues Affecting Minority Participation in Research Studies of Alzheimer Disease." *Alzheimer Disease Associated Disorders* 8 Supplement 4: 38–48.

Whitman, S., Benbow, N. G. Good. 1996. "The Epidemiology of Homicide in Chicago." *Journal of National Medical Association* 88: 781–787.

Williams, David, Yan Yu, and James Jackson. 1997. "Discimination, Race, and Health." Paper presented at the 1997 Joint Meeting of the Public Health Conference on Records and Statistics and Data User's Conference.

Williams, James, T. Saunders, D. Hunt, J. Schorling. 1997. "Prevalence of Coronary Heart Disease Risk Factors among Rural Blacks: A Community-Based Study." *Southern Medical Journal* 90: 814–820.

Wingo, Phyllis, L. Reis, H. Rosenberg, D. Miller and B. Edwards. 1998. "Cancer Incidence and Mortality 1973–1995: A Report Card for the U.S." *Cancer* 82: 1197–1207.

Zambrana, Ruth and Susan Scrimshaw. 1997. "Maternal Psychosocial Factors Associated with Substance Use in Mexican-Origin and African American Low-Income Pregnant Women." *Pediatric Nursing* 23: 253–274.

WEB SITES OF SIGNIFICANCE

Associate Director Office for Minority Health

http://www.cdc.gov/od/adm/

Department of Health and Human Services

http://www.os.dhhs.gov/

National Center for Health Statistics

http://cdc.gov/nchswww/

National Institutes of Health

http://www.nih.gov/

Office of Minority Health

http://www.omhrc.gov/

Chapter 5

African American Alternative Medical Practices

CRITICAL THINKING QUESTIONS

1. Describe your initial perceptions of African American alternative medical practices.

2. Why do African Americans tend to use alternative medicines?

3. What are the major factors that influence the use of alternative medicines?

INTRODUCTION

Alternative medical practices are defined as choices or options of medical care that are not a part of the mainstream or professional health care system. Alternative medical practices include the health values and knowledge, roles, and practices of laypersons, of specialists in folk medicine, and of layperson-specialists such as the vocational practitioners of homeopathic medicine (Aakster 1986).

In the field of medical anthropology, alternative medical practice is referred to as ethnomedicine. Ethnomedicine is defined as how members of a particular cultural and/or ethnic group think about disease/illness and organize themselves toward medical treatment. In general, both terms, ethnomedicine and alternative medical practices, refer to the similar process of seeking medical care that is not a part of the mainstream or professional health care system.

Alternative or ethnomedical therapies are gaining more public attention and are more widely used than most health care professionals may realize (Youngkin and Israel 1996: 39). Champion (1993) stated that in a given year about a third of all American adults use unconventional medical treatments and the 25–49-year age group. These therapies include, but are not limited to megavitamin treatments, relaxation and biofeedback techniques, massage therapy, therapeutic touch, guided imagery, chelation therapy, acupuncture, and herbal medicine (Youngkin and Israel 1996: 39).

The wider usage of alternative therapies encouraged Congress in 1992 to instruct the National Institutes of Health to establishing an Office of Alternative Medicine. The Office of Alternative Medicine provides funding for researchers who want to investigate the efficacy of certain types of alternative medicines. The information learned from all types of research studies on alternative medicines helps the government and the general public to determine which type of alternative medicines is appropriate for the general population. Therefore, the government investigation of alternative medical therapies and the widespread use of alternative medicines indicate that alternative medical therapies are establishing a new and legitimate status in the U.S. health care system (Engebretson and Wardell 1993; Risser and Mazur 1995; Davis and Voegtle 1994; Autotte 1995; Wardwell 1994) .

HISTORY

African Americans are primarily descendants of West African people who share a common history, place of origin, language, food preferences, values, and health beliefs that engender a sense of exclusiveness and self-awareness of being a member of this ethnic group. With regard to health beliefs and health care practices, African Americans are believed to have retained many of the preventive and treatment practices associated with indigenous West African cultures primarily because these methods were perceived to be most useful. Jacques (1976), Jordan (1975), Jackson (1985), Baer (1985), Spector (1985), Goodson (1987), Mbiti (1975), Harvey (1988), Tinling (1967), and Tallant (1990) all contend that African Americans continued to utilize folk and herbal medical practices as a result of the communication difficulties with Europeans and the fears of European physicians.

There is documented evidence that traditional West African health beliefs and herbal remedies were handed down and maintained among various African American populations throughout North America (Spector 1985; Bailey 1991a). For example, oral histories of former slave women from all over the South contained frequent and sometimes elaborate descriptions of the wide variety of plants which constituted the material base from which the slave medical practice operated (Goodson 1987: 200).

Specifically, female African American slave doctors used drugs derived from plants to prevent and cure worms, malaria, croup, pneumonia, colds, teething, and measles. Sometimes, they used the root, and at other times, they selected the leaf, bark, fruit, or gum resin to boil into a tea or make into a poultice or wear in a bag around the neck (Goodson 1987: 200). Not only did African American slave doctors have this medical knowledge of plants, but also many other slaves knew how to diagnose and treat illnesses. In fact, a number of medicine chests have been discovered filled with the popular preparations of the day: calomel, blue mass pills, castor oil, ipecac, tartar emetic, and various tinctures (Ewell 1813). This type of cultural historical information on slave medical health practices illustrates how cultural health practices and beliefs associated with the indigenous West African cultures were shared with the new immigrant, enslaved Africans in America (Postell 1951).

During the 1700s and 1800s in the United States, African American health beliefs and practices continued to show similarities with the West Africans' health beliefs and practices. As more African Americans migrated to northern cities during the Mid-1800s and early 1900s, they carried a repertoire of health care beliefs and practices. African American health beliefs and practices, thus, became a composite, containing elements from a variety of sources: European folklore, Greek classical medicine, modern scientific medicine, vodoun religion, Christianity, and particularly African folklore (Hill 1976). With such a mixture of health belief systems, it is no wonder that African American health beliefs and practices are currently shared by all segments of the American population (Bailey 1991a).

HEALTH

Health is defined as a state of complete physical, mental, and social well-being, not merely the absence of disease, or the ability of an organism to adapt to its environment and circumstances (Green and Ottoson 1994: 699). Although the definitions of health vary from one field to another, the central theme is that health should be viewed holistically—physical and social well-being.

In a study of 21 young African American women between 21 and 40 years of age, Hargrove and Keller (1996) found that these women defined health as avoiding disease and/or illness. In this study, participants described health as a variety of factors and behaviors that assist them in maintaining health or avoiding disease. They also described activities in which they (including family and friends) contribute to good health or assist them in avoiding health problems Many researchers (Bailey 1988; Orque et al. 1983; Leininger 1985; Manuel 1986; Sussman 1988) have found similar definitions of health among other samples of African Americans.

Interestingly, Hargrove and Keller (1996) also found that African American women believed that being "fat or overweight" as an older individual was expected and/or seen as a sign of being healthy; being slim or skinny was looked upon as being sickly (Hargrove and Keller 1996: 7). In this study, it was culturally acceptable to be "slim or skinny" when an individual was younger.

This sample of African American women also believed that it was important that they looked good to the men in their lives. Hargrove and Keller (1996) state that in many cases the women were "heavy, large, and meaty" to please a man. The African American women stated further that obesity or being overweight was descriptive of being healthy, and that obesity was not related to heart disease, hypertension, or diabetes. Eating "healthy" and having enough food to eat were more important to health (8).

Although there is a distinction between good and poor health, African Americans' perception of what constitutes "healthy" encompasses a relatively high tolerance of discomforts from symptoms (Jackson 1981). Studies have shown that African Americans often ignore minor discomforts as backaches, upset stomach, or headaches until they reach such proportions that they interfere with the business of living (Jackson 1981). In fact, African Americans, particularly the elderly, often perceive their health status as "poorer" than do European Americans (Manuel 1986). Furthermore, since one's self-esteem, sanity, and survival are at risk, in a state of health (good or bad), one becomes adaptive, flexible, alert, and able to use a wide range of strategies effectively to endure and reach his/her optimal potential. In other words, until the degree of discomfort impairs daily activities or is acknowledged by the individual's sociocultural network, seeking health care, particularly from mainstream health care facilities, is not warranted.

ILLNESS

Illness is defined as sickness of body or mind; disease is defined as a harmful departure from the normal state of a person or other organism (Green and Ottoson 1994: 697). Often, the public views these two terms similarly. Yet, medical anthropologists and other health care researchers distinguish these two terms as completely different: illness is a subjective abnormality of health, and disease is an objective physiological abnormality.

Illnesses are classified as either naturalistic or personalistic (Snow 1974). Naturalistic agents identify what caused an illness, whereas personalistic agents recognize who caused the illness (Chino and Vollweiler 1986). Such impersonal agents as inadequate rest, poor nutrition, and germs cause illnesses. The etiology of illnesses falls into three general categories: environmental hazards, divine punishment, and impaired sociocultural relationships.

In some cases, serious and life-threatening illnesses are perceived to be sent by God (personalistic agent) or some other personalistic agent as punishment for sin (Snow 1974; Hill 1976). Many African Americans, for example, who suspect a terminal illness may delay medical diagnosis. During this delay and/or denial period, many African Americans turn to powers considered greater than themselves to fathom the reason for the disease, thereby accepting terminal illness as "God's will" and believing that nothing more can be done.

Examples of naturalistic and personalistic causative agents are described in the following two studies. First, a study investigating the treatment patterns of hypertension among 285 African Americans in the Detroit metropolitan area contended that African Americans' beliefs about the etiology of hypertension were based on naturalistic agents (Bailey 1991b). Bailey reported that informants considered inadequate rest, poor nutrition, weather disturbances, and imbalances in hot and cold properties as naturalistic agents affecting their blood pressure. Informants described such "richy" foods as heavily salted greens, pork, and sweets as naturalistic agents. Moreover, cold weather was described as a naturalistic agent that can affect the viscosity of one's blood pressure (294). These findings were directly comparable to those of other studies on folk symptomatology (Blumhagen 1982; Dressler 1982; Garro 1986; Snow 1974).

Second, a study investigating the narratives of 26 African American women with advanced breast cancer found that these women attempted to relate the meanings of their cancer to an indigenous model of health and disease (Mathews, Lannin, Mitchell 1994; Lannin et al. 1998). The women interviewed ranged in age from 39 to 83 years, with the majority being over the age of 50.

Cancer was seen by patients to be the worst of all diseases because they believe it is always fatal and is essentially incurable. Consequently, for many of the women interviewed, cancer resembled illnesses that did not respond to conventional categories or cures in the indigenous medical system (Mathews, Lannin, Mitchell 1994: 795). Thus, the only likelihood of finding a cure for cancer was "to turn it over to God." One of the informants said the following: "Cancer is a horrible disease. It just eats you up. The only one powerful enough to overcome it is the Lord. You just have to trust in Jesus to do battle for you and save you from this horrible affliction" (795). Mathews, Lannin and Mitchell contend that here the battle metaphor is used to portray a struggle between God, as the all-powerful force for good, and cancers as consummate evil.

Mathews, Lannin, and Mitchell stated that another informant had rejected the medical system and its interpretation of the disease primarily because of a bad personal experience with the medical staff and her belief in the causation of the cancer. Fortunately, at the urging of a close friend at the medical center, this informant returned for care under her own terms and guided by her belief in God.

Interestingly, Mathews, Lannin, and Mitchell suggest that too often in the past health care professionals have assumed that patients who delay seeking treatment for cancer or who fail to utilize the screening services available either lack knowledge, are too poor to access services, deny reality, or are excessively fatalistic. In actuality, these patients have well worked out ideas about their own health and about their disease (799). Patients, in this case African Americans, also have well worked out ideas about treatment strategy depending on whether the illness is perceived as naturalistic or personalistic.

TREATMENT ACTIONS: NATURALISTIC CAUSATION

The types and sources of treatment actions among African Americans are likely to vary according to gender, class, region of the United States, and degree of assimilation to mainstream society. In the United States, most ethnic groups have the option of selecting from a variety of sources: (1) formal health professionals; (2) licensed health professionals; (3) alternative or native health practitioners; (4) caregiving network; and (5) self.

If the illness is perceived as naturalistic (i.e., due to inadequate rest, poor nutrition, or germs), African Americans tend to use initially one and/or a combination of the following treatment actions: self-care, caregiving network, alternative (indigenous) health practitioner, and formal health professionals (Jackson 1981; Spector 1985; Jacques 1976; Leininger 1985; Bailey 1991b).

Self-Care

Self-care includes positive steps taken by individuals to either prevent disease or promote general health status through health promotion or lifestyle modification; medical self-care for the identification or treatment of minor symptoms of ill health or self-management of chronic health conditions; and steps taken by laypersons to compensate or adjust for functional limitations affecting routine activities of daily living. National research studies have indicated that African Americans use a variety of self-care strategies depending on the illness and/or disease (Fahie 1998; Becker et al. 1998; Resnicow et al. 1997; Arcury et al. 1996; Skelly et al. 1995; Bailey 1991b).

The use of home remedies or herbs is an example of a self-care strategy. The basic assumption behind the use of herbs/home remedies links the natural organic properties of herbs with the natural healing capabilities of human beings. Herbalists use these organic substances in an effort to neutralize or eliminate one's body of harmful substances that impair its power to heal itself (Lust 1974: 8). According to herbalists, any herb, if mixed and used properly, can treat effectively any natural illness.

Spector (1985) has identified some African American home remedies as successful in the treatment of disease. The following are a few selected examples:

1. A method for treating colds is hot lemon water and honey.
2. When congestion is present in the chest and the person is coughing, the person can be wrapped with warm flannel after his/her chest is rubbed with hot camphorated oil.
3. Hot toddies are used to treat colds and congestion. These drinks consist of hot tea with honey, lemon, peppermint, and a dash of brandy or whatever alcoholic beverage the person likes and has available. Vicks Vaporub is swallowed.
4. Herbs from the woods are used in many ways. Herb teas are prepared to treat pain and reduce fevers. Sassafras tea frequently is used to treat colds.
5. Placing raw onions on the feet and wrapping them in warm blankets can break a fever. (196–197)

In addition, chicken soup is used for a whole host of illnesses. Davis (1997) states that these include upper respiratory illness, lack of energy, the flu, upset stomach, listlessness, fevers, nausea, and vomiting.

In general, self-care strategies such as home remedies and herbs are convenient and effective sources of therapy (Davis 1997). The three major reasons for their continual usage in the African American community are as follows:

1. Folk remedies may be the only alternatives to costly treatment of acute illness by the health care system,
2. Folk remedies have been given the stamp of approval by generations of African American caregivers,
3. The loving care, attention, and overall nurturance that accompanies the use of remedies cannot be overlooked. (433)

Furthermore, Davis (1997) states that employing folk remedies in treatment follows closely the culture of a particular group of people and is replete with memories, comfort, and familiarity. In fact, folk remedies may be so enmeshed in tradition that not to perform them is tantamount to sacrilege. Yet this important understanding may be lacking among health care providers (434).

Caregiving Network

For the purpose of our discussion in this section, I refer to the caregiving network as the lay, nonprofessional, nonspecialist domain of society, where ill health is first recognized and defined, and health care activities are initiated (Helman 1985: 43). It includes all the therapeutic options that people utilize, without consulting either folk healers or medical practitioners. Helman (1985) states that among these options are self-treatment or self-medication; advice or treatment given by a relative, friend, neighbor, or workmate; healing and mutual care activities in a church or self-help group; or consultation with another layperson who has special experience of a particular disorder or of treatment of a physical state.

In reference to African Americans, the caregiving network and the meaning of caregiving are culturally based in long-standing traditions. Health care researchers have also referred to this caregiving network within the African American community as the "informal and/or extended familial network." Whether referred to as informal network, extended familial network or caregiving network, this network consists of those individuals who are family members, friends, neighbors, or other nonfamily associates who would help the individual African American if he or she were sick or disabled (Chatters 1985; Neighbors and Jackson 1984; Chatters et al. 1986; Taylor and Chatters 1986).

Interestingly, this "caregiving network" plays an important social, cultural, and health function in the lives of African Americans (Hayes and Mindel 1973; Stack 1974; Neighbors and Jackson 1984; Haley et al. 1996; Cox and Monk 1996). Neighbors and Jackson (1984) state that social networks are utilized by African Americans as an alternative to formal help seeking as well as a supplement to professional help utilization.

For example, in a national survey of black Americans, Neighbors and Jackson (1984) found that informal help is used more frequently than professional help as a means of coping with problems. Statistics indicated that a vast majority (87%) of the 1,292 African Americans sampled talked to at least one informal helper—most people use informal help (43%) or both informal and formal help (44%). Thus, the majority of respondents were categorized as users of informal help only, even when demographic background and type of personal problem were taken into account (643). In conclusion, Neighbors and Jackson suggest that research on how the social network functions, both as an alternative treatment source and as a referral system should prove to be a fruitful area of investigation for social scientists interested in the help-seeking behavior of African Americans.

Interestingly, the reasons given for caregiving and the high use of the caregiving network among African Americans as it relates to treating illness, again, reflect the importance of cultural values and traditions. For instance, in an in-depth study of seventeen African American caregivers for older ill relatives, Nkongho and Archbold (1995) classified the reasons given for caregiving as: familial, relational, and personal. The familial category consisted of maintaining family integrity and role modeling. Past and present actions affected the relational category, which included reciprocity, affection, and respect. The personal category addressed the caregiver's beliefs, values and attitudes (118). In particular, caregiving among this sample provided a way of demonstrating their beliefs. Beliefs and values identified by caregivers included caring for one's own family and harmony. All (100%) caregivers expressed the importance of looking after, or providing for, their own families. One caregiver stated "You care for your own. You take your sisters and your mama and your daddy and everybody else and you take care of them yourself. You don't need anybody out there taking care of them. It is a thing that you do."

These findings suggest that caregivers and the caregiving network will consistently be an option for seeking care for minor and major illnesses within the African American community.

Alternative Indigenous Health Practitioners

In addition to the caregiving network and the variety of home remedies or patent medicines practiced among African Americans, there are primarily two types of alternative indigenous health practitioners serving the African American community: (1) independent practitioner and (2) cultic practitioner (Baer 1985: 327). These two types of alternative indigenous health practitioners operate as individuals or are affiliated with some sort of occult supply store, either as the owner, an employee, or someone who rents office space. The cultic practitioner is affiliated with a religious group and practices in both public and private settings. The multiplicity of African American alternative indigenous health practitioners today stems from the role adaptability of traditional African American healers of the past (Bailey 1991a).

For instance, one type of African American alternative indigenous health practitioner, the neighborhood prophet/Old Lady, does not dispense medicine but merely advises clients about concocting herbal medicines. Rather than selling or giving an herbal remedy, the Old Lady tells the client to use it in varying proportions to treat the perceived illness. In addition, she gives advice for various emotional, personal, and domestic problems. She does not receive monetary gifts for her service, only gifts of food or expression of gratitude (Jordan 1979: 38). The neighborhood prophet/Old Lady treats the individual's mind, body, and spirit in an attempt to return the individual to harmony with nature.

This alternative indigenous alternative health practitioner as well as many others have successfully matched their holistic approach in treating illness/disease with the model or perception of treating illness/disease among many African Americans. Although there are no specific utilization data to document the total numbers of African Americans seeking care from these alternative indigenous health practitioners, their presence and growth within the alternative health delivery network cannot be denied and overlooked anymore.

Formal Health Practitioners

In this section, formal health practitioners are referred to as licensed medical doctors (M.D.'s) and D.O.' s (doctors of osteopathic medicine) in licensed allopathic (M.D.–staffed) and osteopathic hospitals. The U.S. Department of Health and Human Services (1986) regularly documents the number of physician contacts by the general public. Interestingly, the national health care utilization data have always showed a distinctive difference between African Americans' and European Americans' use of formal health practitioners. For example, blacks sought care from the doctor's office less (47%) than did whites (57.7%). Blacks were also less likely to contact a doctor by phone (9.2%) than were whites (13.4%). Yet, blacks were reported to have experienced more physician contact in hospital outpatient departments (21.4%) than whites (13.7%) and to have more physician contact at home (5.8%) than whites (2.5%) (U.S. Department of Health and Human Services 1986).

Most health care researchers would contend that an obvious explanation for the difference of physician utilization between blacks and whites is economics. There is no doubt that the costs of seeking care and the lack of health insurance cause many African Americans to delay or not seek care from formal health practitioners. However, some researchers contend that are other social and cultural factors have truly caused the disparity in seeking care from formal health practitioners.

In particular, Blendon's et al. (1989) study of 10,130 persons living in the continental United States found that even blacks above the poverty line have less access to medical care than their white counterparts. The researchers contend that ethnic-related differences in health care arrangements and lifestyle were the most significant factors in disparity between black and white health care utilization.

For example, blacks are more likely than whites to report that during their last visit their physician did not inquire sufficiently about pain, did not tell them how long it would take for prescribed medicine to work, did not explain the seriousness of the illness or injury, and did not discuss tests or examination findings. In addition, fewer than three-fifths of blacks were completely satisfied with the care provided during their last hospitalization, compared with over three-fourths of whites (Blendon et al. 1989). It is apparent that there are differences not only in access but also in the perception of the care provided for blacks and whites. Blacks seem to adhere to ethnomedical beliefs and practices, and they use alternative health care therapies more extensively than do whites (Blendon et al. 1989).

Treatment Actions: Unnatural Causation

Unnatural illnesses are perceived to be caused by a supernatural spirit, magic, sorcery, voodoo or some other personalistic agent (Snow 1974; Hill 1976; Bailey 1991a). The literature on African American illness causation suggests that the African American healing tradition considers the universe a place where the forces of good and evil, God and Satan, struggle for control (Gregg and Curry 1994: 522). Therefore, unnatural illnesses are perceived to be a struggle between the forces of good and evil.

Within this belief system, religion or spirituality is of most importance to illness perceived to be caused by unnatural means. Even though religion and spirituality are most commonly reported as important sources of social support for African Americans, they can also be used for dealing with unnatural illnesses in a more positive way (Stolley and Koenig 1997; Gregg and Curry 1994; Ford et al. 1998; Jackson and Nixon 1970; Taylor and Chatters 1986). Taylor and Chatters (1986) and Stolley and Koenig (1997) and many other researchers have shown that African Americans' use of religion and spirituality for natural as well as unnatural illnesses is their particular method of treating an illness/disease within their health belief system.

Another means of treating an unnatural illness and sometimes natural illness is with voodoo "rooting." As a form of religion, voodoo is a complex of African belief and ritual governing, in large measure, the religious life of African natives (Jordan 1975). Harvey (1988) states that "as a belief system which combined historical conceptions with practices that were acceptable in a hostile social environment, voodoo is a striking example of a cultural adaptive mechanism used by members of an oppressed group as a survival technique." The African American form of voodoo medicine consists of three components.

The first is the mystic component, which deals with the supernatural such as spells and spirits. The second component is that part of voodoo that deals with psychological support of the individual, and the third part is herbal and folk medicine. African American voodoo prospers particularly in the South, primarily because it fills a void left by inaccess and denial of medical care by formal American health practitioners (Jordan 1979: 38).

An example of its usage was indicated in a study by Morgan (1996). Examining the prenatal care patterns of African American women in selected U.S. urban and rural cities, she found that one of her key informants first denied believing in voodoo but on a subsequent visit gave an account of her experience of having a spell on her. Additionally, this key informant as well as others believed that unnatural illnesses demand alternative indigenous healers and practices for relief. Morgan stated that in both settings, alternative indigenous health care providers were often found to ameliorate or cure natural and unnatural illnesses and other misfortunes that befell African Americans.

In conclusion, African Americans tend to consult an alternative indigenous health practitioners primarily because of:

1. their attempt to cope with health problems within the context of one's resources and social and cultural environment;
2. their belief that alternative indigenous health practitioners have some control over the forces that cause illness/diseases in a person's life, whereas Westernized medical physicians cannot heal certain cases of illness and misfortune and;
3. lower monetary expense associated with such treatments (Cockerham 1986: 88; Hill 1976: 14).

CONCLUSION

This review of the alternative medical practices among African Americans highlights the "cultural basis" for its continual use and status within the African American community. The persistence of traditional African American health beliefs and practices provides a meaningful alternative to mainstream formal medicine for many African Americans because of its role in maintaining a sense of ethnic identity. It also indicates a pattern of adaptation to social and economic conditions both within the African American community and in the larger society.

According to surgeon general David Satcher (1992), "the knowledge, attitudes, and behavior of African Americans must be targeted and enhanced in order to close the health gap as we know it." Once we recognize and understand the framework of the multitude of factors that influence African American health care beliefs and practices, increased adherence to such health care issues as hypertension, cerebrovascular diseases, diabetes, HIV/AIDS, prenatal care, and cancer educational outreach programs can finally be improved.

POST-EVALUATION QUESTIONS:

1. Describe the cultural historical factors that influenced the use of African American alternative medical practices among African Americans.

2. What is the theoretical basis for causation of various illnesses according to African American alternative health belief system?

3. What should a health care professional do when he or she recognizes that an African American patient uses alternative medicines?

REFERENCES

Aakster, C. W. 1986. "Concepts in Alternative Medicine." *Social Science and Medicine* 22: 265–273.

Arcury, T., S. Bernard, J. Jordan, and H. Cook. 1996. "Gender and Ethnic Differences in Alternative and Conventional Arthritis Remedy Use Among Community-Dwelling Rural Adults with Arthritis." *Arthritis Care and Research* 9: 384–390.

Autotte, P. 1995. "Folk Medicine." *Archives Pediatric Adolescence Medicine* 149: 949–950.

Baer, Hans. 1985. "Toward a Systematic Typology of Black Folk Healers." *Phylon* 43: 327–343.

Bailey, Eric. 1988. "An Ethnomedical Analysis of Hypertension among Detroit Afro-Americans." *Journal of the National Medical Association* 80: 1105–1112

———. 1991a. *Urban African American Health Care*. Lanham, MD: University Press of America.

———. 1991b. "Hypertension: An Analysis of Detroit African American Health Care Treatment Patterns." *Human Organization* 50: 287–296.

Becker, G., Y. Beyene, E. Newsom, and D. Rodgers. 1998. "Knowledge and Care of Chronic Illness in Three Ethnic Minority Groups." *Family Medicine* 30: 173–178.

Benner, Patricia and Judith Wrubel. 1989. *The Primacy of Caring: Stress and Coping in Health and Illness*. New York: Addison-Wesley.

Berry, Mary and John Blassingame. 1982. *Long Memory: The Black Experience in America*. New York: Oxford University Press.

Blendon, R., L. Aiken, H. Freeman, and C. Correy. 1989. "Access to Medical Care for Black and White Americans." *Journal of American Medical Association* 261: 278–281.

Blumhagen, Dan. 1982. "The Meaning of Hypertension." In *Clinically Applied Anthropology*. N. Chrisman and T. Maretzki. eds. Pp. 297–324. Boston: D. Reidel Publishing.

Braithwaite, Ronald and Sandra Taylor eds. 1992. *Health Issues in the Black Community*. San Francisco: Jossey-Bass.

Champion, E. 1993. "Why Unconventional Medicine in the United States." *New England Journal of Medicine* 328: 282–283.

Chatters, Linda, Robert Taylor and James Jackson. 1985. "Size and Composition of the Informal Helper Networks of Elderly Blacks." *Journal of Gerontology* 40: 605–614.

———. 1986. "Aged Blacks' Choices for an Informal Helper Network." *Journal of Gerontology* 41: 94–100.

Chino, Harriet and Lothar Vollweiler. 1986. "Etiological Beliefs of Middle-Income Anglo Americans Seeking Clinical Help." *Human Organization* 45: 245–254.

Chrisman, Noel. 1977. "The Health Seeking Process: An Approach to the Natural History of Illness." *Culture and Medical Psychiatry* 1: 351–377.

Cockerham, William. 1986. *Medical Sociology.* Englewood Cliffs, NJ: Prentice-Hall.

Cox, Carole and Abraham Monk. 1996. "Strain among Caregivers: Comparing the Experiences of African American and Hispanic Caregivers of Alzheimer's Relatives." *International Journal of Aging and Human Development* 43: 93–105.

Crosby J. et al. 1981. *The African Experience in Community Development.* Reynoldsburg, OH: Advocate Publishing Group.

Davis, Ruth. 1997. "Understanding Ethnic Women's Experiences with Pharmacopeia." *Health Care for Women International* 18: 425–437.

Davis, B. and K. Voegtle. 1994. *Culturally Competent Health Care for Adolescents: A Guide for Primary Care Providers.* Chicago, IL: American Medical Association.

Dressler, William. 1982. *Hypertension and Culture Change: Acculturation and Disease in the West Indies.* New York: Redgrave Publishing.

Editorial. 1995. "Folk Medicine." *Archives Pediatric Adolescent Medicine* 149: 949–950.

Eisenberg D., R. Kessler, C. Foster, F. Norlock, D. Calkins, and T. Delbanco. 1993. "Unconventional Medicine in the United States." *New England Journal of Medicine* 328: 246–252.

Engebretson, Joan and Diane Wardell. 1993. "A Contemporary View of Alternative Healing Modalities." *Nurse Practitioner* 18: 51–55.

Ewell, J. 1813. *Planter's and Mariners' Medical Companion.* Philadelphia, PA: Scholarly Press.

Fahie, V. 1998. "Utilization of Folk/Family Remedies by Community-Residing African American Elders." *Journal of Cultural Diversity* 5: 19–22.

Ford, Marvella, Barbara Tilley and Patricia McDonald. 1998. "Social Support among African American Adults with Diabetes, Part 2: A Review." *Journal of the National Medical Association* 90: 425–432.

Franklin, John and Alfred Moss. 1988. *From Slavery to Freedom: A History of Negro Americans.* New York: Alfred A. Knopf.

Garro, Lynda. 1986. *"Cultural Models of High Blood Pressure."* Paper Presented at the 85th American Anthropological Association. Philadelphia, PA.

Goodson, Martia. 1987 "Medical-Botanical Contributions of African Slave Women to American Medicine." *The Western Journal of Black Studies* 2: 198–203.

Green, Lawrence and Judith Ottoson. 1994. *Community Health.* Seventh Edition. St. Louis: Mosby.

Gregg, J. and R. Curry. 1994. "Explanatory Models for Cancer among African American Women at Two Atlanta Neighborhood Health Centers: The Implications for a Cancer Screening Program." *Social Science and Medicine* 39: 519–526.

Griffith, Ezra et al. 1984. "An Analysis of the Therapeutic Elements in a Black Church Service." *Hospital and Community Psychiatry* 35: 464–468.

Haley, William, D. Roth, M. Coleton, G. Ford, C. West, R. Collins and T. Isobe. 1996. "Appraisal, Coping, and Social Support as Mediators of Well-Being in Black and White Family Caregivers of Patients with Alzheimer's Disease." *Journal of Consulting and Clinical Psychology* 64: 121–129.

Harding, Vincent. 1981. *There Is a River: The Black Struggle for Freedom in America.* New York: Vintage Books.

Hargrove, Hazel and Colleen Keller. 1996. "Young Black Women: Defining Health." *Journal of the National Black Nurses Association* 3–14.

Harrison, Ira and Diana Harrison. 1971. "The Black Family Experience and Health Behavior." In *Health and the Family: A Medical-Sociological Analysis.* Charles O. Crawford ed. Pp. 175–199. New York: Macmillan.

Harvey, William. 1988. "Voodoo and Santeria: Traditional Healing Techniques in Haiti and Cuba." In *Modern and Traditional Health Care in Developing Societies.* Christine Zeichner, ed. Pp. 101–114. New York: University Press of America..

Harwood, Alan. 1981. *Ethnicity and Medical Care.* Cambridge: Harvard University Press.

Hayes, W. and C. Mindel. 1973. "Extended Kinship Relations in Black and White Families." *Journal of Marriage and the Family.* 35: 51–57.

Helman, Cecil. 1985. *Culture, Health and Illness.* Bristol: Wright.

Hill, Carole. 1976. "Folk Medical Belief System in American South: Some Practical Considerations." *Southern Medicine* 11–17.

Hines, Paulette and Nancy Boyd-Franklin. 1982. "Black Families." In *Ethnicity and Family Therapy.* M. McGoldrich and J. Pearce, eds. Pp. 84–107. New York: The Guildford Press.

Horner, Ronnie, E. Oddone, and D. Mathar. 1995. "Theories Explaining Racial Differences in the Utilization of Diagnostic and Therapeutic Procedures for Cerebrovascular Disease." *The Milbank Quarterly* 73: 443–462.

Hurley, D. 1995. "Pharmacists Need to Increase Knowledge of Herbal Remedies as Use Skyrockets." *Pharmacy Practice News* (May): 24–25.

Jackson, Jacquelyne. 1981. "Urban Black Americans." In *Ethnicity and Medical Care*. A. Harwood, ed. Pp. 37–129. Cambridge, MA: Harvard University Press.

———. 1985. "Race, National Origin, Ethnicity, and Aging." In *Handbook of Aging and the Social Sciences*. Robert Binstock and Ethel Shanas, eds. Pp. 264–303. New York: Van Nostrand.

———. 1991. *Life in Black America*. New York: Sage.

Jackson, Jacquelyne. Jackson, Oscar and Waldense Nixon. 1970. "Medicine in the Black Community." *California Medicine* 113: 57–61.

Jacques, Gladys. 1976. "Cultural Health Traditions: A Black Perspective." In *Providing Safe Nursing Care for Ethnic People of Color*. Marie Branch and Phyllis Paxton, eds. Pp. 115–123. New York: Appleton-Century Crofts.

Jordan, Wilbert. 1975. "Voodoo Medicine." In *Textbook of Black-Related Diseases*. Richard Williams, ed. Pp. 716–738. New York: McGraw-Hill.

———. 1979. "The Roots and Practice of Voodoo Medicine in America." *Urban Health* 8: 38–41.

Lannin, D., H. Mathews, J. Mitchell, M. Swanson, F. Swanson, and M. Edwards. 1998. "Influence of Socioeconomic and Cultural Factors on Racial Differences in Late-Stage Presentation of Breast Cancer." *Journal of the American Medical Association* 279: 1801–1807.

Leininger, Madeleine. 1985. "Southern Rural Black and White American Lifeways with Focus on Care and Health Phenomena." In *Qualitative Research Methods in Nursing*. Madeleine Leininger, ed. Pp. 195–216. New York: Grune and Stratton.

Lust, John. 1974. *The Herb Book*. New York: Bantam Books.

Manuel, Ron. 1985. "Demographics and the Black Elderly." Paper Presented at the Gerontological Meetings. Chicago. Illinois.

Marwick, C. 1992. "Congress Wants Alternative Therapies Studied; NIH Responds with Programs." *Journal of the American Medical Association* 268: 957–958.

Mathews, H., D. Lannin, and J. Mitchell. 1994. "Coming to Terms with Advanced Breast Cancer: Black Women's Narratives from Eastern North Carolina." *Social Science and Medicine* 38: 789–800.

Mbiti, John. 1975. *Introduction to African Religion*. Ibadan: Institute for Urban Studies.

Morgan, Marjorie. 1996. "Prenatal Care of African American Women in Selected USA Urban and Rural Cultural Contexts." *Journal of Transcultural Nursing* 7: 3–9.

Neighbors, Harold and James Jackson. 1984. "The Use of Informal and Formal Help: Four Patterns of Illness Behavior in the Black Community." *American Journal of Community Psychology* 12: 629–644.

Nkongho, Ngozi and Patricia Archbold. 1995. "Reasons for Caregiving in African American Families." *Journal of Cultural Diversity* 2: 116–123.

Orgue, Modesta, B. Bloch, and L. Monroy. 1983. *Ethnic Nursing Care: A Multicultural Approach.* St. Louis: The C.V. Mosby.

Postell, William. 1951. *The Health of Slaves on Southern Plantations.* Baton Rouge, LA: Louisiana State University Press.

Resnicow, K., R. Vaughan, R. Futterman, R. Weston, J. Royce, C. Parms, M Hearn, M. Smith, H. Freeman, and M. Orlandi. 1997. "A Self-Help Smoking Cessation Program for Inner-City African Americans: Results from the Harlem Health Connection Project." *Health Education and Behavior* 24: 201–217.

Risser, A. and L. Mazur. 1995. "Use of Folk Remedies in a Hispanic Population." *Archives Pediatric Adolescence Medicine* 149: 978–981.

Satcher, David. 1992. "Afterwords." In *Health Issues in the Black Community.* Ronald Braithwaite and Susan Taylor, eds. San Francisco: Jossey-Bass.

Saunders, Elijah. 1991. *Cardiovascular Diseases in Blacks.* Philadelphia: F. A. Davis Company.

Skelly, A., J. Marshall, B. Haughey, P. Davis, and R. Dunford. 1995. "Self-Efficacy and Confidence in Outcomes as Determinants of Self-Care Practices in Inner-City, African American Women with Non-insulin Dependent Diabetes." *Diabetes Educator.* 21: 38–46.

Snow, Loudell. 1974. "Folk Medical Beliefs and Their Implications for Care of Patients." *Annals of Internal Medicine* 81: 82–96.

———. 1977. "Popular Medicine in a Black Neighborhood." In *Ethnic Medicine in the Southwest.* Edward Spicer, ed. Tucson, AZ: University of Arizona Press.

Spector, Rachel. 1985. *Cultural Diversity in Health and Illness.* New York: Appleton-Century Crofts.

Stack, Carol. 1974. *All Our Kin: Strategies for Survival in a Black Community.* New York: Harper & Row.

Staples, Robert. 1971. "Towards a Sociology of the Black Family: A Theoretical and Methodological Assessment." *Journal of Marriage and Family* 33: 19–138.

Stolley, Jacqueline and Harold Koenig. 1997. "Religion/Spirituality and Health among Elderly African Americans and Hispanics." *Journal of Psychosocial Nursing* 35: 32–38.

Sussman, L. 1988. "Treatment Seeking for Depression by Black and White Americans." *Social Science and Medicine* 24: 187–197.

Tallant, Robert. 1990. *Voodoo in New Orleans.* Gretna, LA: Pelican.

Taylor, Robert. 1985. "The Extended Family as a Source of Support to Elderly Blacks." *The Gerontologist* 25: 488–495.

Taylor, Robert and Linda Chatters. 1986a. "Patterns of Informal Support to Elderly Black Adults: Family, Friends, and Church Members." *Social Work* 432–438.

————. 1986b. "Church-Based Informal Support among Elderly Blacks."
    The Gerontologist 26: 637–643.
Tinling, David. 1967. "Voodoo, Root Work, and Medicine." *Psychosomatic
    Medicine* 29: 483–490.
U. S. Department of Health and Human Services. 1986. *Black and Minority
    Health: Report of the Secretary's Task Force: IV*. Washington DC:
    U.S. Government Printing Office.
Wardwell, Walter. 1994. "Alternative Medicine in the United States." *Social
    Science and Medicine* 38: 1061–1068.
Warren, Rueben. 1992. "Health Education and Black Health Status." In *Health
    Issues in the Black Community*. Ronald Braithwaite and Susan Taylor,
    eds. Pp. 241–254. San Francisco: Jossey-Bass..
Williams, Richard Allen. 1975. *Textbook of Black-Related Disease*; New York:
    McGraw-Hill.
Youngkin, Ellis and Debra Israel. 1996. "A Review and Critique of Common
    Herbal Alternative Therapies." *Nurse Practitioner* 21: 39–45.

WEB SITES OF SIGNIFICANCE

Office of Minority Health Resource Center

http://www.omhrc.gov

National Center for Complementary and Alternative Medicine

http://altmed.od.nih.gov/nccam

Black Health Net

http://www.blackhealthnet.com

Healthweb African American Health

http://www.lib.mus.edu/health/hw/minority/african.html

Part III

How To Do Medical Anthropological Fieldwork

In general, medical anthropological fieldwork involves observing, listening, asking questions, analyzing, and summarizing patients'and/or health care professionals' thoughts and behaviors as they relate to a specific and/or general health care or medical issue. A step-by-step approach to medical anthropological fieldwork is described for the first time student, researcher, practitioner, and the general public. Qualitative methods such as participant observation, focus groups, and in-depth interviews are emphasized. The procedure for completing a medical anthropological fieldwork project consists of four phases: (1) preparing and adapting to the field; (2) medical anthropological fieldwork techniques; (3) ethnographic fieldwork data analyses; and (4) reflective comments. In addition, ethical issues of research as they relate to an African American researcher are discussed.

Chapter 6

Strategies for Applied Medical Anthropology Health Care Research

CRITICAL THINKING QUESTIONS

1. What are the particular strategies for conducting applied medical anthropology health research?

2. Are there any particular advantages in conducting an applied medical anthropology health research study?

3. What can nonanthropologists learn from using applied medical anthropology health research strategies?

INTRODUCTION

Ethnographic research has a long and continuing history in cultural anthropology to investigate human behavior. To understand and to describe a cultural and/or ethnic group, anthropologists engage in ethnographic fieldwork. *Fieldwork* refers to firsthand observation of human societies—as a means of gathering data and testing hypotheses generated by theories. This means living with people, eating their food, learning their language, listening to gossip, examining the items they produce, asking questions, recording answers, and, above all, simply watching the people's daily routines and interactions. Those who conduct this type of research are referred to as ethnographers.

Ethnographers study how people live and how they communicate and interact with one another. Material and nonmaterial goods are of interest to the eth-
nographer, as are the folktales, symbols, rituals, and expressive arts (Leininger
1985a: 36). As ethnographers pay close attention to how people live, social
structural features such as politics, religion, kinship, education, and technology
become apparent to the researchers. Thus, a general ethnographic study is the
principal means for obtaining a holistic view or total perspective of people in
their physical and sociocultural environments (Leininger 1985a; Spradley and
McCurdy 1972; and Spradley 1980).

The use of ethnographic methods in the health care field continues to open
new doors of opportunity for applied medical anthropologists. Yet, bringing the
new and growing awareness of health professionals closer to ongoing and expanding applied medical anthropology and the use of ethnographic methods is
more likely to occur if we can show that anthropology can make a cost-effective
contribution (Chrisman and Maretzki 1982). The continuing challenge is to
build bridges between the clinical and public health fields with the applied
medical anthropology field. Kleinman (1980), Fabrega (1974), Eisenberg
(1977), Leininger (1978), and Schreiber and Scrimshaw (1979) are considered
as the early bridge builders who pioneered the fields of medicine, nursing, and
public health with anthropology.

For example, in the field of public health, ethnographic methods such as the
Rapid Assessment Procedures (RAP) have been used to address a variety of
public health problems. Rapid assessment procedures are ethnographic methods
for quickly gathering social, cultural, and behavioral information relevant to
specific health-related problems and prevention programs (Harris, Jerome, and
Fawcett 1997: 375). RAP has been used to solve problems with the World
Health Organization Global Program on AIDS (Scrimshaw et al. 1991), agricultural public health issues of northeast Thailand (Subhadhira et al. 1988), and
other international health programs. Distinguishing features of RAP include

1. formation of a multidisciplinary research team, including a member indigenous to the cultural group of interest,
2. development of materials to train indigenous team members,
3. use of several data collection methods to verify information through triangulation,
4. iterative data collection and analysis to facilitate continuous adjustment, and
5. completion of the project quickly, usually in four to six weeks. (Harris,
   Jerome, and Fawcett 1997: 375).

Ethnographic techniques used in RAP include in-depth key informant interviews, behavioral observation, and focus groups (Manderson and Aaby 1992;
Scrimshaw and Hurtado 1987). Data generated from the RAP are analyzed using standard techniques developed for qualitative data, including content analysis and ethnoclassifications (Pelto and Pelto 1987; Scrimshaw et al. 1991).
Internal validity and reliability of conclusions drawn from RAP are strengthened
through triangulation (using multiple team members and/or research methods to

gather similar data). Data are compared to verify both the accuracy of information and conclusions that are drawn (Harris, Jerome, and Fawcett 1997: 376).

In a community-based public health initiative, Braithwaite, Bianhi, and Taylor (1994) discovered that the rapid ethnographic assessment procedures proved effective in documenting community health concerns and in providing data for people of color and their participation in coalition partnerships. This community-based initiative involved two local health departments, a medical school, a school of public health, and three communities (two suburban and one innercity). Needs assessment profile reports served to educate indigenous citizens about their communities and to provide them with information to make or argue a point with agency policymakers (412). In summary, the ethnographic techniques were the integral tool for galvanizing and mobilizing communities for social action relative to generating a health promotion and disease prevention agenda.

In the clinical setting, ethnographic methods have been shown to be very effective in better understanding a patient's illness perception. In particular, Blumhagen (1982), who explored some of the illness beliefs of mainstream Americans attending an outpatient clinic at the Seattle Veteran's Administration, found that the use of the explanatory model interview helped to facilitate communication between practitioner and patients.

A nineteen-item semistructured interview schedule based on Kleinman's explanatory model questions (Kleinman 1980) was developed and pretested on six individuals who were not part of the study (Blumhagen 1982:304). Blumhagen (1982) revised the interview schedule and administered it to 117 patients in the clinic. He found the following:

A knowledge of what the popular beliefs are around a common illness condition can lead to more intelligent questioning. Thus, for example, a person with hypertension could be asked "Some people think that nervousness is associated with this illness. How do you see that applying to yourself?" A person who was delivering a biomedical model can sometimes be shifted to a deeper, more significant layer of illness belief explication by this type of question. (316)

Thus, by using the ethnographic method such as the explanatory model interviews can lead to improved patient adherence.

The following sections describe the applied medical anthropological strategies that I used for my particular applied medical anthropological studies.

PREPARING AND ADAPTING TO THE FIELD

In any fieldwork project, the first issue is the "topic" of the project. That is, the researcher should "brainstorm" for a period of time about potential topics of the project. This brainstorming process consists of developing a list of at least ten potential projects and determining whether the project will be descriptive, explanatory, or exploratory. Once the researcher arrives at a conclusion in this area, the project can progress to the second stage of preparing and adapting to the field.

This stage involves background research of your topic: conducting preliminary research in a variety of outlets such as library research, newspaper and magazine articles, Internet Web sites and news groups, and personal connections to the focus of the study. The primary purpose of conducting background research is twofold: (1) to reduce the researcher's culture shock and (2) to recognize one's personal biases.

Culture shock is an event that places the health researcher in an uneasy situation in which he or she feels uncomfortable, nervous, anxious, and embarrassed. The health researcher feels this way primarily because of unfamiliarity with the cultural patterns of informants. If some type of background research is completed prior to conducting the field research, then the health care researcher can be better prepared for the encounters in the field.

Second, once health researchers truly admit their own biases to themselves and to others, then a better understanding of their informants' health care issues can be appreciated. Thus recognizing their biases helps health researchers realize their own personal preferences to certain health care issues and helps them move closer to the role of "objective" health researchers.

The third step of preparing and adapting to the field is called the *researcher's effect*. It is critical for health researchers to be aware that their presence in the field may affect the behavior of their informants. In order not to change the behavior or information shared among informants, health researchers must try to be as inconspicuous as possible when collecting field data. Sitting off to the side or staying out of the direct line of sight when informants are sharing detailed information may help when collecting field data. Thus, when preparing to collect field data, it is significantly important to plan ahead on how and where the health researchers will situate themselves.

The fourth and final step of preparing and adapting to the field is referred to as *ideal versus real cultural patterning*. Before reaching the field and before collecting field data, the health researcher will often encounter from key informants' "ideal" standards or views of their health cultural pattern. The ideal cultural pattern is what people say they do, yet in fact it is often different from what they really do. It is crucial for the health researcher to recognize the difference of what people say versus what they really do. In other words, people will complete surveys and participate in focus group sessions and say that they practice a certain health care pattern, yet they actually practice an alternative health care pattern. For the health researcher, determining the difference between "ideal versus real" cultural patterning is of critical importance to the foundation of every applied medical anthropology study.

MEDICAL ANTHROPOLOGICAL FIELDWORK TECHNIQUES

In the field of anthropology, one element that has remained constant throughout its history is the use of qualitative methods to collect field data. Distinguished scholars such as Hurston (1942; 1995), Boas (1928; 1943), Malinowski (1929; 1954), and Kluckhohn and Murray (1954) and Mead (1928; 1955) established the foundations for qualitative research methods. Their early fieldwork studies among provided the framework for qualitative research in the future.

Qualitative research refers to the methods and techniques of observing, documenting, analyzing, and interpreting attributes, patterns, characteristics, and meanings of specific contextual features of the phenomenon under study (Leininger 1985a: 5). Leininger states that with this research method, the focus is on identifying the qualitative features, characteristics, or attributes that make the phenomenon what it is. This includes documenting and fully describing major features of the phenomenon such as human events, life situations, health care issues, and other aspects under study. In general, the use of qualitative methods helps to discover cultural health patterns, to witness the actions of informants/clients, and to understand the informants/clients' perspective.

Observation

The first two phases of qualitative research are observation and participant observation. These phases are particularly important to any qualitative health care project primarily because they allow the researcher to view the health care problem from a uniquely insightful perspective.

Often, observation has been taken for granted. As most anthropologists recognize, observation is the key to any quality fieldwork project. Critically observing behavior of individuals or interactions between health care professionals and patients provides an opportunity to witness the "real cultural" patterning that exists. Whether the observation is of a waiting room of an outpatient clinic, or the interaction of a nurse practitioner with a patient who needs special assistance because of a disability, the reactions of patients to each other in a busy emergency room clinic, or a free public health fair, observation is a significant research tool in providing the researcher "direct evidence" of a health problem.

Leininger (1985a) states that the researcher obtains a broad view of the situation and gradually makes detailed observations. Allowing some time to make detailed and documented observations is essential before interacting or participating more directly with the people because it permits the researcher to establish what is occurring before influencing the situation as a participant. It also permits the people some time to observe the researcher at a distance and to "size up" his or her behavior as a stranger (53). Thus, researchers who use observation as a research tool must develop their own particular style and approach.

Health researchers need to become aware of their own strengths and weaknesses in observational style. Pelto and Pelto (1978) state that one should practice observing and recording events in order to discover observational biases and to develop more systematic techniques of recall. One should find out how extensive notetaking must be in order to ensure accuracy of recall. One must learn to direct attention to features that tend to be neglected (70). Thus, the key to successful critical observation is *practice, practice,* and *practice.*

Participant Observation

The second most important phase to a qualitative health research project is participant observation. Participant observation is a method by which an observer maintains a presence in a health care situation for the purpose of scientific investigation (Fitzpatrick 1981). The observer participates in the daily life of the people under study, either openly in the role of researcher or covertly in some disguised role, observing things that happen, listening to what is said, and questioning people over some length of time (Becker and Geer 1957: 28). By participating, the researcher learns from the people and feels, experiences, and learns by direct involvement in activities (Leininger 1985a).

For example, my participant observation as a volunteer in the Hypertension Clinic of Henry Ford Hospital in Detroit (Chapter 9) provided me an opportunity to feel and to experience what it was like to be a part of the staff at a major urban hospital (Photo 6.1). A majority of the people with whom I worked treated me as though I was a regular staff member. Although they knew that I was a doctoral student at Wayne State University and conducting a study on patients' health beliefs as they relate to hypertension, I obtained a degree of acceptance with the hospital culture and a better appreciation of those who work in clinical hospital settings. Therefore, using participant observation can significantly enlighten the health researcher on a number of social and cultural health issues that were often neglected.

Informants

Through participant observation, the health researcher notes which persons are most involved in the actions—they are usually the ones with the greatest amount of firsthand information—they are referred to as "informants" (Pelto and Pelto 1978: 74). Working with informants is the hallmark of ethnographic fieldwork. It involves an ongoing relationship (Spradley and McCurdy 1972: 41).

The "informant" plays a vital role for the health care researcher. Informants are representatives of the cultural and ethnic group and who show potential to reveal substantive data on the domain of study (Leininger 1985b:47).

Photo 6.1
Participant Observation at Henry Ford Hospital (Detroit, Michigan 1984)

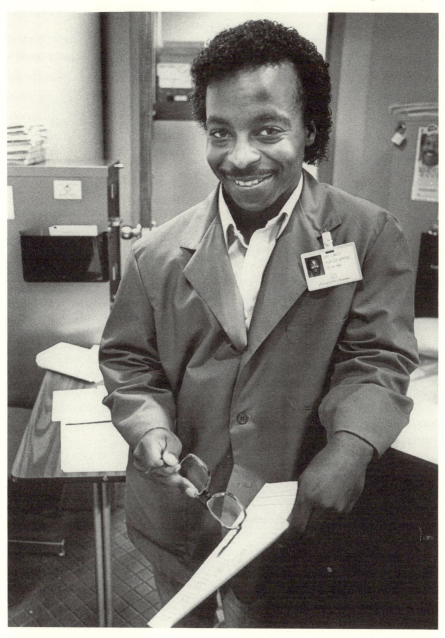

Informants are different from "respondents." Informants provide descriptions of the group or research setting as a whole whereas respondents provide the investigator with personal accounts—what they thought, saw, and did during some event or about some issue. Fitzpatrick (1978); Spradley (1979) and Spradley and McCurdy (1972) state that in many ways informants can be thought of as narrators, knowledgeable about the setting and its actors, who provide the researcher with insight into what is going on. Informants, therefore, are the spokespersons for the group about any particular health care issue in the community.

Type of Interviews

Generally, there are three types of interviews. The first type is called informal or open-ended interviews (Bailey 1982; Leininger 1985b; and Spradley and McCurdy 1978). Informal interviews are ideal to elicit *emic* (insider's perspective) data and get "inside the head" or obtain the worldview thoughts and experiences of the informant (Leininger 1985b: 54). Leininger (1985b) states it is truly an art and skill for the interviewer to listen actively and patiently after posing an open-ended question to the interviewee.

The second type of interview is semistructured interview, which is a combination of both informal and structured types. It is designed to elicit both definitive and unexpected kinds of information from the interviewee (Leininger 1985b:55).

The third type of interview is the structured interview, designed to elicit specific responses to specific questions. This type of interview is more often used to control responses to fit specific variables and to ask the same questions of all sampled individuals. Examples of structured questions are, How many times have you used the local health clinic? or How many times did you participate in prenatal health care classes before the birth of your child?

With each interview strategy, there are obvious advantages and disadvantages. For instance, the advantages of using structured interviews are as follows:

1. They are standardizable;
2. They provide a frame of reference;
3. They clarify dimensions of concepts; and
4. They allow less chance for interviewer variability. (Wagenaar 1981)

Although these advantages provide the researcher with quantitative results and well-defined, categorical findings, structured interviews have a number of disadvantages:

1. They may force statement of opinion even when informant knows nothing about the topic;
2. The researcher may overlook a possible alternative; and

3. The informants may make different interpretations of the questions. (Wagenaar 1981)

Informal interviews or unstructured interviews involve a number of advantages and disadvantages. As stated earlier, informal interviews are much like a casual conversation between the researcher and the informants. The casualness and flexibility of the interview allows the researcher to ask many more in-depth and personal questions.

The major advantages of using informal/unstructured interviews are as follows:

1. They provide better indicators of whether informant is telling the truth or knows what he or she is talking about.
2. They are appropriate for intensive study of attitudes.
3. They suggest hypotheses.
4. They clarify response alternatives, and
5. They allow data to emerge—grounded theory at work. (Wagenaar 1981)

Although the advantages of using informal interviews may outweigh the disadvantages, there are two areas of concern: (1) analysis difficult is and costly, and (2) comparability is difficult (Wagenaar 1981). Often these two issues influence many health researchers to opt for a different and more structured style of interviewing.

As stated earlier, semistructured interviews combine the informal and structured interview approaches. That is, semistructured interviews elicit specific, categorical responses from the informants but also include opportunities for the informants to elaborate on as many concepts or issues as they desire. Therefore, the semistructured interviewing approach is best for the researcher who requires categorical, quantitative data and insightful, in-depth qualitative data.

Focus Group Interviews

Focus group interviews are a qualitative research method that provides rich data on dynamic attitudes of individuals interacting in a group about a designated topic. Focus group methodology uses a standardized series of questions to elicit individual responses within the context of a group. This method benefits from both group interaction and group dynamics. In this environment, participant responses include the interplay of group members, which allows for greater depth of response, social context, and emotion. In addition, focus groups allow the researcher to hear directly from participants, using their own vocabulary, language, and communication patterns—essential components when working with differing ethnic and cultural groups.

The focus group leader participates to guide the group in addressing the inquiry topic of cultural attitudes and values that the group has about the specific health care topic. The group leader also provides further feedback concerning group interaction.

An ideal focus group leader is comfortable and familiar with group process and is able to exert a mild, yet unobtrusive, control over the participants (Nyamathi and Shuler 1990: 1285). Moreover, the focus group leader must be able to communicate clearly and be adequately knowledgeable about the topic of conversation. It is critical that the focus group leader manages a fine line between following the focus group questions, to assure that the purpose and objectives for the group will be achieved, and maintaining group enthusiasm and interest (Nyamathi and Shuler 1990: 1285).

Focus Group Studies

The use of focus groups in gathering qualitative health data on various segments of the African American population continues to be a new area of enlightenment for health care researchers. Specifically, a number of focus group studies have been very effective in researching critical health care issues in the African American population. For instance, Nyamathi and Shuler (1990) used focus group interviews to develop a culturally sensitive AIDS education program for African American women. As part of a larger study designed to provide counseling and HIV testing for the at-risk group, African American women who were (1) homeless, (2) intravenous drug users (IVDU) or sexual partners of IVDUs, (3) diagnosed with a sexually transmitted disease, or (4) prostitutes were invited to participate. The women participated in six focus groups. All groups were held in private rooms in one of two homeless or one of two drug rehabilitation programs (1286).

All sessions were conducted by two African American nurse researchers who were thoroughly trained to provide guidance and direction. All women who participated in the focus groups and signed informed consent received ten dollars at the completion of the two hour session (Nyamathi and Shuler 1990: 1286). A sample of 66 African American women who participated in the six focus groups ranged in age from 18 to 68; 64 (97%) were under 50 years of age.

The focus group qualitative data suggested that in order to provide useful assistance, health care professionals need to fully understand the concerns and stresses these women experience and attempt to devise strategies that enhance feelings of control. By assisting the women's active participation in seeking resources needed resources, an element of control may be maintained. A thorough assessment should include the individual's perception of the situation and the needs experienced. More importantly, an assessment of how their needs can be met without usurping control from the client is imperative (Nyamathi and Schuler 1990: 1287). In general, Nyamathi and Schuler contend that the qualitative information obtained from the use of focus groups has been invaluable in tailoring an education program to the needs of a select population.

Focus group methodology was also used to ascertain answers to the issue of what cultural barriers impact African American women's participation in breast and cervical cancer screening. Williams, Abbott, and Taylor (1997) conducted three focus group sessions consisting of a total of 32 African American women from Flint, Michigan. Most of these women were older than 45 years (51%); single, divorced, or widowed (69%); had a high school education or better (65%); reported household incomes of $20,000 or less (66%) and were employed (47%) (48). Transcripts were analyzed for trends and themes that emerged as a result of the questions asked.

Williams, Abbott, and Taylor (1997) stated that the results of the focus group discussions with low-income African American women indicate that intensive recruitment efforts were needed to increase utilization of breast cancer screening services. Interpersonal contacts such as telephone calls reminding them of regular checkups and transportation to doctor's offices were two methods of encouraging preventive care, thereby making these women feel that hospitals were caring places and that the women were not just another face in the health facility (54). Focus group discussion with African American women also indicated that health promotion messages should be culturally sensitive and acknowledge the role of spirituality in their lives.

Finally, Williams, Abbott, and Taylor (1997) stated that focus group discussions provided important information that would not have been obtained through telephone surveys or personal interviews. In fact, they stated, "The group dynamics created an atmosphere where many ideas and feelings were expressed that would not have come out if participants had been interviewed individually" (55).

Focus group methodology was also used to gather qualitative data in recruiting African American women at risk for noninsulin-dependent diabetes mellitus into exercise protocols (Carter-Nolan, Adams-Campbell; and Williams 1996). Five of the focus groups comprised of 39 African American women less than 45years (mean age: 27.9). The remaining focus group comprised 18 African American women more than 45 years (mean age: 50.9 years). The mean age for all 57 women was 34.6 years. Content was analyzed within each group, and ranges of attitudes, beliefs, and barriers were determined across all groups.

Carter-Nolan, Adams-Campbell, and Williams (1996) found that several barriers toward physical activity exist and tend to be more prominent in the African American population. The barriers included low income, safety concerns, time management, low motivation, lack of social support, and accessibility of exercise facilities. Addressing these barriers, the researchers contend that this will prove beneficial in increasing the likelihood of African American women's participating in exercise protocols. Moreover with regard to the advantage of the focus group methodology, the researchers suggested that it was a useful technique for reaching minority populations:

Focus groups may be used to increase participation of black women in physical activity programs because: 1) the women share a common problem and are more likely to discuss it openly with each other and 2) the women, with consistent encouragement from the moderator, will have a sense of ownership of the solutions being provided. (561)

Finally, focus group methodology was used to assess attitudes associated with the willingness of African Americans to participate in prostate cancer clinical trials. Robinson, Ashley and Haynes (1996) conducted focus group sessions among 46 men, 40 years of age and older, in south central Los Angeles. The sessions were moderated by an African American research team and all sessions were audiotaped for transcription, then analyzed with the assistance of the Ethnograph Qualitative Analysis Program.

Robinson, Ashley, and Haynes found the following qualitative results:

Most stated that they would be willing to participate in prostate cancer clinical trials. Many preferred entering a trial that was conducted at a black facility. They would want to know if the hospital had enough funds to conduct the trials. They would request information about the track record of the medical center's research activities. (83)

In addition, these researchers found that the focus group data revealed that major obstacles to entering prostate cancer clinical trials were the lingering memories of the Tuskegee trials, lack of trust of the medical establishment and fear of adverse reaction to the experimental drug or therapy. Moreover, too much monetary compensation would increase concerns with respect to the safety of the experimental protocol (83). In general, Robinson, Ashley, and Haynes felt that their study will be invaluable in laying the foundation for future investigations and interventions aimed at increasing participation of minorities in clinical trials.

Focus Group Procedures & Guidelines

Focus group sessions vary with each research topic. However, there are general procedures and guidelines for focus group sessions. For researchers who are unfamiliar with the procedures and guidelines for conducting focus group interviews and for those researchers who want the best results, the following points are suggested:

Preparing for the Focus Group

1. Review the questions the day of or several hours before the focus group session.
2. Practice asking the questions to a friend or a colleague before the focus group session.
3. Determine where and how to arrange the seating for the focus group session.
4. Arrange the seating in a semicircular or full circle fashion (depending upon the number of participants).
5. Establish the best place to arrange the audio and videotape in the room (Usually off to the side or out-of-the-way of participants).

6. Review the questions again with the local community facilitator (key informant).
7. Bring refreshments to the focus group sessions.
8. As participants arrive, introduce yourself to them and invite them to have some refreshments. (This helps to establish immediate rapport.)
9. Be patient to start the focus group session. (Allow 5 to 15 minutes for individuals to arrive at designated time of focus group session.)

Conducting the Focus Group

1. At the start of the focus group session, welcome all participants and state the general purpose of the study.
2. Allow participants to ask as many questions as possible about the study.
3. After all questions are answered, restate that there are no right or wrong answers and that "we are here to learn from you."
4. Pose the first focus group question.
5. If one person responds, encourage others to share their story.
6. If several individuals respond, encourage a one-at-a-time discussion.
7. Learn to respect each response from all participants.
8. Ask for clarification for terms or phrases not familiar to you (Can you explain that term further?).
9. Do not demean or talk down to any participants regardless of their vocabulary or speech pattern.
10. Ask for assistance from your community facilitator to keep the conversation at a steady pace.
11. Keep long elaborate examples to a minimum. (Some participants may want to share very long cases with the group. Tell them that you would want to hear these cases after the session).
12. Focus group questions do not have to be asked consecutively (Allow for flexibility, and the flow of the focus group will determine which questions to ask accordingly).
13. Keep your biases and opinions to yourself! (This allows for participants to speak freely on very critical topics.)
14. After the final focus group question is answered, thank the participants again and restate what will happen to their answers.
15. Assure all participants that they can receive a copy of the study's results when completed.

Individual In-Depth Profiles

The individual in-depth profile is a special way of obtaining individuals' ideas and experiences from their particular viewpoint. The individual in-depth profile yields insightful information that is usually not obtainable by the structured questionnaire or the group setting of a focus group. Questions such as the following are examples of the individual, in-depth profile investigation that I used.

1. I would like to hear your view on what it's like to be an African American in this country and how you believe that your home setting and cultural values have helped (or hindered) you in successfully living a quality life,
2. If you could do it all over again, what stage of your life would you have changed since living here in this area?

In general, the purposes of the individual in-depth profiles are (1) to obtain intimate and detailed knowledge about the person; (2) to gain a comprehensive view of the individual's sociocultural environment and lifestyle; and (3) to generalize from the individual to the rest of the particular cultural and/or ethnic group. For those researchers who are unfamiliar with the procedure and questions and for those researchers who want the best results from individual in-depth interview session, the following points are suggested:

Procedure for Individual In-depth Profiles

1. Practice asking the questions to a friend or a colleague before the individual in-depth interview session.
2. The individual in-depth interview session should be arranged immediately after a focus group session or entirely separately from the session.
3. Ask the community key informant (facilitator) who would be a good candidate to participate in the individual in-depth interview.
4. Select at least two potential individuals (of those who participate in a focus group) for the individual in-depth interview (male/female).
5. As the facilitator discusses the format of the focus group session with community residents, ask for volunteers to participate in a one-on-one, individual in-depth interview session following the focus group session or arrange a special time to meet.
6. Once the individual in-depth volunteer is selected, discuss with the individual the goals of the individual in-depth interview.
7. Answer as many questions as possible pertaining to the purpose of the individual in-depth interview.
8. Once the session begins, maintain a relaxed and informal atmosphere.
9. The facilitator can determine how long (minutes/hours) the individual in-depth session will last.
10. Always tape-record the session in order to recall detailed information shared with you.
11. Always ask for clarity of key cultural terms or meanings of words/phrases.
12. Always thank the individual for sharing such important information with you in order to understand their point of view.

Types of General Individual In-depth Questions

1. Could you please share with me a little bit about yourself? (probe–current lifestyle situation)
2. Let's talk about where you were born and what you remember about your early days/years of growing up. (probe–family patterns, community, and childhood experiences).
3. I would like to hear your view on what it's like to be an African American growing up in this area and your experiences or your family's in seeking health care. (probe–cultural adaptation to the local health care system)
4. I would like to hear your general thoughts on keeping yourself well or healthy. (probe–cultural practices of preventive therapy)
5. Have you or any of your family members used the local health care system for your current health problem? What was it like? probe–specific health care incidents).
6. Have you or any of your family members used the local health care system for any other type of care? What was it like (probe–differences of emergency care vs preventive care)
7. I would like to hear your thoughts on how you would improve the local health care system as it relates to your community. Are there any improvements that need to be made, or is the local system fair to all people? (probe–perception of health care system to local community)

Sampling

One of the most often asked questions when conducting applied medical anthropological research are, how many people should be a part of my study, and what particular group should I study? The response is, what is your topic? You can have as many or as few people as you want in your study. This is the advantage of conducting applied medical anthropological research. Although applied medical anthropological studies are more flexible in research design than other fields of study, there are a number of commonalities. Sampling is one of these commonalities.

Four type of sampling procedures often used in applied medical anthropological studies. They are: (1) random, (2) stratified, (3) convenience, and (4) snowball. Depending on factors such as funding, time schedule, and design of the study, the researcher has the option to use one or several of the sampling procedures.

Bailey (1978) describes the sampling procedures as follows:

1. Random—each person in the universe has an equal probability of being chosen for the sample.
2. Stratified—separating the population into non-overlapping groups, called strata, then selecting a simple random sample from within each stratum.

3.   Convenience—the researcher chooses the informants by chance.
4.   Snowball—the researcher meets and interviews key informants who in turn selects other key informants (91–100).

Each sampling procedure has its advantages and disadvantages to the study. The researcher must determine to what degree the advantages outweigh the disadvantages in using a certain sampling procedure.

Ethnographic Fieldwork Data Analyses

Depending on the type of ethnographic fieldwork method used, health researchers have the option to analyze their data through either or both qualitative or quantitative approaches. In each case, health researchers' major objective is to reduce or to "make sense" of all the observations and interviewing that they completed during the study. Analyzing data, whether quantitative (statistics) or qualitative (words), can be one of the most difficult and confusing stages or one of the easiest stages of the study.

Quantitative Analyses

In all of my studies, I have selected the easiest and least complicated approach in analyzing my field data. Often, I have had to utilize basic quantitative analyses with basic qualitative analyses in order to obtain a "balance" of the information being gathered.

For example, statistics are a tool for understanding data. The purpose of statistical analyses is to reduce data to some manageable form so that conclusions of various sorts can be drawn (Wagenaar 1981: 281). I have used basic statistical analyses for establishing a "foundation of consistency of information" gathered from my informants. Standard parametric statistics such as t-test, Pearson correlations, and multiple regressions may provide results to highlight similarities or differences between groups being compared. Whether these comparative statistical data support or disprove a hypothesis, they provide me with additional evidence to support the qualitative findings.

Qualitative Analyses

Simply put, qualitative data are categories or labels that describe a behavior, action, thought, or group of people. Categories are an invention of ways to classify and organize experience (Spradley and McCurdy 1972: 61). Basically, the use of qualitative data analyses helps the researcher to classify and to organize the observations and interviews into specific "categories."

Although there are a wide array of qualitative data analyses used, such as content analyses, ethnoscience analysis, grounded theory analysis, componential analysis, symbolic analysis, and structural functional analysis, I have used primarily four different analyses:

1. ethnographic data,
2. life history profile,
3. individual in-depth, and
4. thematic and pattern. (Leininger 1985b)

Ethnographic Method

The ethnographic method of analysis primarily focuses on the use of ethnographic (emic) cultural data obtained directly from the people, through mainly the participant observation method (Leininger 1985b: 58). The method includes also *etic* (outsiders perspective) and other generational observational data obtained while studying people over a short or long period of time (Leininger 1985: 58).

Life History Analyses

The life history method focuses on analyzing normal and abnormal life history events, patterns, and their relationship to health maintenance. This method helps to identify longitudinal patterns of living related to wellness, caring, health care seeking, and sociocultural barriers of the health care system (Leininger 1985b: 64).

Individual In-Depth Analyses

The individual in-depth analysis focuses on a particular individual's mode of maintaining health, patterned illness, or other styles of survival through long (or short) spans of time in different (or the same) environmental contexts. This method of analysis is important to:

1. obtain intimate and detailed knowledge about the individual;
2. identify health, care, and illness patterns;
3. identify actual and potential factors leading to illness; and
4. gain a comprehensive view of the individual's environment and lifestyle over short or long periods of time. (Leininger 1985: 64)

Theme and Pattern Analyses

Theme and pattern analysis focuses on the analysis of different cognitive and identifiable themes and patterns of living or of behavior. Raw data are analyzed by identifying and bringing together components or fragments of ideas or experiences, which often are meaningless when viewed alone. Patterns are generally small units of behavior that contribute to themes. Themes are large units of analysis derived from patterns which can explain multiple aspects of human behavior (Leininger 1985b: 60–61).

In summary, each of these qualitative data analyses attempts to synthesize the words, actions, and behaviors into simple categories of meanings.

Reflective Comments

Reflective comments "look back" thoughtfully on what happened to recapture the situation and total process of what happened and how the people responded to you, the researcher (Leininger 1985b: 53). Leininger (1985b) stated that understanding what transpired between researcher and the people being studied is essential to get an accurate and full account of the situation or event. Reflective comments provide the researcher with direct and immediate interpretation of the particular site visit or key informant interview. After leaving the field, it is especially important for researchers to document immediately their reflective comments in their fieldwork notebook. These reflective comments, thoughts, and feelings actually start the process of qualitative analysis primarily because they help the researcher to focus on certain categories of behavior.

In other words, if the researcher uses theme and pattern qualitative analysis, the themes and patterns of the particular group or individual begin to formulate in the thought processes of the individual researcher. Once the actual qualitative analysis of the data begins, the researcher will already have developed categories of cultural domain, thereby making the qualitative analysis much easier and more understandable.

ETHICS OF HEALTH CARE RESEARCH: PERSON OF COLOR ISSUES

In any research, past and present, there is always an array of ethical issues one must attempt to follow. Depending on the topic, the institution, or area of the country, ethical guidelines of health care research are a matrix of mass confusion. When studying people of color, such as African Americans, there are additional ethical issues to follow.

As an African American health care researcher, I have been told for approximately fifteen years that there are two major disadvantages in studying your own people: (1) objectivity will be compromised, and (2) subjectivity to informants will influence data findings. From graduate school to my position as an associate professor, these ethical issues have always been brought to my attention. Both of these research issues are legitimate ethical statements that can affect the outcome of any research, particularly when an African American is studying his or her own ethnic population.

However, the aforementioned disadvantages are far outweighed by the advantages. I contend that being an African American and conducting health care research on African Americans have allowed me to see, feel, experience, and analyze health care data (qualitatively and quantitatively) in a more "in-depth" way than my non-African American health care researchers. The specific advantages are as follows:

1. Understanding cultural sensitivity health care issues;
2. Developing rapport and trust at an early stage of the research project;
3. Understanding past discriminatory health care issues and their effects on African American perceptions and health seeking;
4. Recognizing my role as an "ethnic cultural broker"—a person of color who has obtained trust from the community and trust from the health care system;
5. Attempting to make applied health care projects "ethically" responsible for the community being studied.

For example, in Chapter 11, my collaboration with the Houston Health Department challenged my "ethnic culture broker" role. On one hand, I was a part of the department in the role of chairperson and organizer of a local health fair, and, on the other hand, I was a representative of the local African American community because of the rapport and trust that I had developed through my extensive fieldwork in the community. I therefore interacted between two cultural groups while also addressing two major health and sociopolitical problems. Since there were a number of serious health problems that the local African American community needed to address, I implemented a variety of culturally competent strategies to encourage the community residents to take health care action.

Second, I had to resolve a number of sociopolitical problems with the local advisory board in an effort to design this health screening program in a culturally competent way. Thus, I used my "ethnic culture broker" role as a major advantage in empowering the local African American community to take action on their health care problems and in empowering the local advisory board in changing the policy of health care intervention for communities of color.

To reiterate, there are more advantages than disadvantages in being a person of color (African American) who studies the applied medical anthropological issues related to African Americans. The data gathered by African American researchers often provide an in-depth perspective into the qualitative cultural health and social issues associated with the African American population.

Nonetheless, one must be cautious and not assume that all African American researchers are best suited to study the African American population. Some African American researchers may have no connection to the African American community. Moreover, some African American researchers may not desire to focus any of their health care research studies on the African American population. It is often assumed by non-African American and African American researchers that all African American researchers (persons of color) are naturally adept to research African American health issues. In other words, just because you're an African American does not mean that you automatically relate to the African American community. Although there are definite advantages in being an African American medical anthropologist and conducting research on African Americans, health care research has more to do with the individual—not his or her ethnicity.

CONCLUSION

Medical anthropological research strategies provide health care researchers and clinicians with an additional tool to learn more about the populations they research and serve (Hazuda 1997). As discussed in this chapter, qualitative research offers all those who learn how to do it effectively an opportunity to learn not only more about their clientele, their research subjects, but also more about themselves. The added advantage of qualitative research is that it allows us to truly appreciate the in-depth, innermost feelings an individual has about his or her particular health problem. Once more health care researchers and clinicians incorporate qualitative research strategies into their practice, then perhaps more answers than questions will be solved with regard to patient care and patient adherence.

POST-EVALUATION QUESTIONS

1. Discuss which applied medical anthropological research strategies you would select for your study.

2. Which qualitative strategy appears to be most utilized for researching in the African American population?

3. Discuss the advantages of using qualitative research strategies in the clinical and public health setting.

4. Describe and explain additional ethical issues that a person of color may encounter when conducting applied medical anthropological research.

REFERENCES

Bailey, Kenneth. 1982. *Methods of Social Research*. 2nd ed. New York: Free Press.

Becker, Howard S. and Blanche Geer.1957. "Participant Observation and Interviewing: A Comparison." *Human Organization* 16: 28–32.

Blumhagen, Dan. 1982. "The Meaning of Hypertension." In *Clinically Applied Anthropology: Anthropologists in Health Science Settings*. Noel Chrisman and Thomas Maretzki. eds. Pp. 297–324. Boston: D. Reidel,

Boas, Franz. 1928. *Anthropology and Modern Life*. New York: Norton.

Boehm, Susan and Patricia Coleman-Burns et al. 1995. "Prostate Cancer in African American Men: Increasing Knowledge and Self-Efficacy." *Journal of Community Health Nursing* 12(3): 161–169.

Braithwaite, Ronald, Cynthia Bianhi, and Sandra Taylor. 1994. "Ethnographic Approach to Community Organization and Health Empowerment." *Health Education Quarterly* 21(3): 407–416.

Carey, James. 1993. "Linking Qualitative and Quantitative Methods: Integrating Cultural Factors into Public Health." *Qualitative Health Research* 3 (3): 298–318.

Carter-Nolan, Pamela, Lucille Adams-Campbell and Jerome Williams. 1996. "Recruitment Strategies for Black Women at Risk for Noninsulin-Dependent Diabetes Mellitus into Exercise Protocols: A Qualitative Assessment." *Journal of National Medical Association* 88(9): 558–562.

Chrisman, Noel and Thomas Maretzki. eds. 1982. *Clinically Applied Anthropology: Anthropologists in Health Science Settings*. Boston: D. Reidel.

Crane, Julia and Michael Angrosino. 1992. *Field Projects in Anthropology. A Student Handbook*. Prospect Heights, IL: Waveland Press.

Dignan, Mark and Patricia Carr. 1992. *Program Planning for Health Education and Promotion*. 2nd ed. Philadelphia: Lea and Febiger.

Eisenberg, Leon. 1977. "Disease and Illness." *Culture, Medicine, and Psychiatry* 1. 1: 9–23.

Fabrega, Horacio. 1974. *Disease and Social Behavior*. Cambridge: MIT Press.

Fitzpatrick, John.1981 "Reflections on Being a Complete Participant."in *Readings for Social Research*. ed. Theodore Wagenaar. Belmont: Wadsworth, Pp. 118–129.

Harris, Kari, Jerome, Norge and Stephen Fawcett. 1997. "Rapid Assessment Procedures: A Review and Critique." *Human Organization* 56:3: 375–378.

Hazuda, Helen. 1997. "Minority Issues in Alzheimer Disease Outcomes Research.." *Alzheimer Disease and Associated Disorders* 11:6: 156–161.

Hurston, Zora Neale. 1942. *Dust Tracks on a Road*. Philadelphia: Lippincott.

———. 1995. *Folklore, Memoirs, and Other Writings: Mules and Men; Tell my Horse; Dust Tracks on a Road; Selected Articles*. New York: Library of America.

Kleinman, Arthur. 1980. *Patients and Healers in the Context of Culture*. Berkeley: University of California Press.

Kluckhohn, Clyde and H. Murray. 1954. *Personality in Nature, Society, and Culture*. Second ed. New York: Knopf.

Knafl, Kathleen et al. 1988. "Blending Qualitative and Quantitative Approaches to Instrument Development and Data Collection." *Journal of Professional Nursing*. January-February 30–37.

Kutsche, Paul. 1998. *Field Ethnography: A Manual for Doing Cultural Anthropology*. Upper Saddle River, NJ: Prentice-Hall.

Leininger, Madeleine. 1978. *Transcultural Nursing: Concepts, Theories, and Practices*. New York: John Wiley.

———. 1985a. *Qualitative Research Methods in Nursing*. New York: Grune and Stratton.

———. 1985b. "Ethnography and Ethnonursing: Models and Modes of Qualitative Data Analysis." In *Qualitative Research Methods in Nursing*. Madeleine Leininger, ed. Pp. 33–72. New York: Grune and Stratton.

Malinowski, Bronislaw. 1929. "Practical Anthropology." *Africa* 2: 23–38.

———. 1954. *The Science of Culture and Other Essays*. Garden City, NJ: Anchor Books.

Manderson, Lenore and Peter Aaby. 1992. "An Epidemic in the Field? Rapid Assessment Procedures and Health Research." *Social Science & Medicine* 35: 7: 839–850.

Mead, Margaret. 1928. *Coming of Age in Samoa*. New York: William Morrow.

———. 1955. "Effects of Anthropological Field Work Models on Interdisciplinary Communication in the Study of National Character." *Journal of Social Issues* 11: 3–11.

Nyamathi, Adeline and Pam Shuler. 1990. "Focus Group Interview: A Research Technique for Informed Nursing Practice." *Journal of Advanced Nursing* 15: 1281–1288.

Pelto, Pertti and Gretel Pelto. 1978. *Anthropological Research: The Structure of Inquiry*. Second ed. New York: Cambridge University Press.

Robinson, S.., M. Ashley, M. and M. Haynes. 1996. "Attitude of African-Americans Regarding Prostate Cancer Clinical Trials." *Journal of Community Health* 21: 77–87.

Schreiber, Janet M., and Scrimshaw, Susan C. M. 1979. "Anthropologists in Schools of Public Health." *Medical Anthropology* 3:3: 309–338.

Scrimshaw, Susan and E. Hurtado. 1987. *Rapid Assessment Procedures for Nutrition and Primary Health: Anthropological Approaches to Programme Improvement*. Published jointly by the UCLA Latin American Center, the United Nations University (Tokyo) and UNICEF.

Scrimshaw, Susan, M. Carballo, L. Ramos, and B. Blair. 1991. "The AIDS Rapid Anthropological Assessment Procedures: A Tool for Health Education Planning and Evaluation." *Health Education Quarterly* 18(1): 111–123.

Spradley, James and David McCurdy. 1972. *The Cultural Experience. Ethnography in Complex Society*. Prospect Heights, IL: Waveland Press.

Spradley, James. 1979. *The Ethnographic Interview*. New York: Holt, Rinehart and Winston.

————. 1980. *Participant Observation*. New York: Holt, Rinehart and Winston.

Subhadhira,S., Simaraks S., and Lovelace, G.W. 1988. "Introduction." In *Rapid Rural Appraisal in Northeast Thailand. Case Studies.* Lovelace G.W., Subhadhira S. and Simaraks S., eds. Pp. 3–19. KKU-Ford Rural Systems Research Project, Khon Kaen University, Khon Kaen,

Wagenaar, Theodore. 1981. *Readings for Social Research*. Belmont, California: Wadsworth.

————. 1981. "Social Statistics Without Formulas."In *Readings for Social Research.* Theodore Wagenaar, ed. Pp. 281–301. Belmont, CA: Wadsworth Company.

Williams, G., Roderic Abbott, and D. Taylor. 1997. "Using Focus Group Methodology to Develop Breast Cancer Screening Programs that Recruit African American Women." *Journal of Community Health* 22 (1): 45–56.

WEB SITES OF SIGNIFICANCE

Society for Applied Anthropology

http://www.telepath.com/sfaa

The Qualitative Report

http://nova.edu/ssss/QR/index.html

Part IV

Medical Anthropology Case Studies: Clinic, Community and Public Health Settings

The following medical anthropological case studies highlight the different types of fieldwork strategies used for a medical anthropological project and show how the author gradually developed his particular style of research. Studies took place in clinic, community, and public health settings located in Ohio, Michigan, Indiana, Texas, and Georgia.

Chapter 7

Fieldwork in a
Cardiopulmonary Clinic

CRITICAL THINKING QUESTIONS

1. Why is it important to conduct fieldwork in a hospital?

2. How are cultural issues related to health care in this clinic setting?

3. What can the medical anthropologist do to assist health care professionals in a clinical setting for African Americans?

INTRODUCTION

Fieldwork in a clinical setting is challenging and provides the basis for an important perspective in health research. This research project was primarily a study designed to describe the relationship between the health practitioner and the patient at a cardiopulmonary site. An additional focus of this research project was to examine to what degree black lung disease affects the quality of life and health status of African American patients. The project consisted of analyzing three components:

1. The compliance rate of the patient to scheduled physical examinations and interview sessions;
2. The relationship between physician and technician; and
3. The communication between health practitioner and patient.

Upon completion of analyzing the ethnographic data, a familiar issue became apparent: What is the value of a medical anthropologist in a clinical setting? The medical anthropologist must strive to introduce sociocultural and ethnocultural health issues to the biomedical world in a cost-effective method.

This fieldwork project was designed to collect only qualitative data from observing interactions between health care professionals and African American patients at a cardiopulmonary clinic. The fieldwork was conducted from June to August 1983 in a major hospital located in Cincinnati, Ohio.

BACKGROUND INFORMATION

Occupational medicine is defined by health problems that are caused by, or that interfere with, one crucial aspect of society—work (Cullen 1998: 12). The basic principles of occupational medicine are diverse: to promote the health and productivity of workers; to prevent injuries and illnesses that may interfere with work, to treat as effectively as possible those who may be harmed by work, and to rehabilitate the sick and injured to return to work or to the highest level of functioning possible (Cullen 1998: 12).

This applied medical anthropological fieldwork project concentrated on the last function of occupational medicine—to diagnose, treat, and rehabilitate the sick for their return to work. Those who were diagnosed as "sick" in this study were those individuals who suffered from black lung disease, asthma, and/or other chronic obstructive lung disease.

The term "black lung" is a nonmedical term referring to an aggregation of respiratory complaints, including asthma, chronic bronchitis, and emphysema, in coal miners (Brooks et al. 1995: 292; Last 1998). Patients diagnosed with black lung, asthma, or other chronic obstructive lung disease were referred to this clinic for treatment.

PHASE 1: PREPARING AND ADAPTING TO THE FIELD

To begin this fieldwork project, I telephoned local hospitals to find out if there were any opportunities for volunteering in a specific clinic where I could see patient and doctor interaction. After several calls and refusals from a few hospitals, I received an open invitation from one hospital, "Hospital B." After approval from the staff, I was scheduled for the grand tour of the clinic, and the staff assigned me to the cardiopulmonary clinic.

Once I learned that the cardiopulmonary clinic was to be the place for my fieldwork project, I began to research the topic "cardiopulmonary." I visited the campus library and researched the topic. The topic was foreign to me so I researched journal articles and books. After reviewing all the significant research articles, books, and materials from the campus library, I began to feel more comfortable with the topic, yet I still was unsure about how to conduct this fieldwork project.

During the day of my scheduled tour, I arrived at the hospital early. To familiarize myself with the hospital, I checked in at the volunteer's desk and took a personal tour by myself. I walked from one department to another, observing every aspect of the hospital environment. In particular, I focused on the interactions of patients with the staff, doctors, and nurses. Although my personal tour through the hospital was brief, I began to get a feel for the atmosphere of the hospital and an idea that patients of all walks of life received a multitude of health care services at the various clinics in this hospital.

Once I arrived at the clinic, I met the nurse assigned to coordinate my activities in the clinic. After introductions and general overview of the clinic's operations, she gave me a tour of the clinic and the nearby departments of the hospital. Initially, my nurse informant talked only about the general procedure of the hospital activities. Later, as our tour ended, she began to share more detailed insights on the clinic's daily activities. Interestingly, the information that I gathered from this very first day through observation and informal discussion helped me become oriented to the hospital and clinic and, in particular, helped me to begin to understand the "culture" of this biomedical setting.

The clinic consisted of four major sections: (1) pulmonary services, (2) cardiac rehabilitation services, (3) cardiac stress testing services, and (4) black lung services. Each section has the same number of offices.

PHASE 2: MEDICAL ANTHROPOLOGY FIELDWORK TECHNIQUES

Initially, I used only observation as a means of gathering qualitative data. Within a week, I used participant observation to collect my preliminary fieldwork data. I spent many of my participant observations in two sections— the black lung clinic and the cardiac stress testing area.   My participant observation activities included volunteering as a file clerk in the clinic. My responsibilities consisted of cataloging and filing patients' records. After completing my volunteering activities, I was free to interact with the clinic staff and patients.

I collected my qualitative fieldwork data by observing 21 physical examinations. Additionally, I conducted 35 semistructured interviews with patients and health practitioner informants. The health practitioner informants consisted of the pulmonary technician, the cardiac technician, and the coordinator of the clinic.

Visits to the clinic lasted approximately four hours, twice a week in the afternoons. During each visit, I observed four health assessment interviews between the patient and the health practitioner. I also observed two cardiac stress tests during each session. Immediately after the interaction between the patient and health practitioner, I recorded my observations. I did the same after each of the interviews that I conducted at the clinic.

PHASE 3: ETHNOGRAPHIC FIELDWORK DATA ANALYSES

In general, patients who received treatment at the cardiopulmonary clinic were elderly adults (50–75 years), 25% of whom were black, and 75% of whom were white. Males outnumbered females 9 to 1, and a majority of the patients resided in the surrounding Appalachian regions. According to my nurse informant, the clinic's patient population was reflective of those who needed care in the community.

The black lung clinic and the cardiac stress testing service were two sections of the cardiopulmonary clinic that were of interest to me. In particular, the black lung clinic diagnoses and rehabilitates any working or retired coal miner who experiences black lung disease and/or related respiratory ailments. Miners who apply to the program and meet the admission criteria undergo a clinical assessment to determine the extent of their disease. If a miner qualifies for rehabilitation, the individual receives a physical examination. Next, the clinic admits the individual to the rehabilitation program and groups all males with other miners who have similar disabilities. The rehabilitation (rehab) program consists of three classes, one a week for three consecutive weeks. The classes are designed to teach the patients basic anatomy, physiology, and breathing exercises.

The cardiac stress testing service is located in the center of the cardiopulmonary clinic. In this room, the equipment consists of a treadmill, an electrosphygmomanometer, an oxygen saturation machine, a heart rate machine, skin electrode hookups, and a couch.

My cardiac technician informant informed me that cardiac stress testing or exercise electrocardiography is an integral tool in the clinical evaluation and management of patients with suspected or known cardiovascular disease. It is commonly used as a screening procedure for normal subjects thought to be at risk of ischemic heart disease. Currently, the motor-driven treadmill or the electrically braked bicycle erogometer with various multistage exercise protocols has become the accepted and standardized method of exercise (stress) testing.

Observation Analyses: Cardiac Stress Testing

During the administration of the cardiac stress test, I observed two significant qualitative issues concerning the informed consent statement and the interactions between the patient and physician. For example, before each stress test, the clinic requires a patient to sign an informed consent statement. This is a major protocol of the clinic.

On this particular occasion, the cardiac technician forgot to obtain the patient's signature for the informed consent statement. Once the oversight was recognized, the technicians held a conference and decided to explain the predicament to the patient and then give him the option of signing the informed consent statement. The patient agreed and signed the statement, thereby clearing the technician of any possible litigation action.

The importance of this event illustrated the "team effort" concept that was often conveyed to me throughout my fieldwork. From the very first day upon entering this clinical setting, the medical staff insisted that the "team effort" approach was the major reason for the success of this cardiopulmonary clinic. This concept of "team effort" became a major "code of ethics" to follow when the staff was placed in difficult decision-making situations.

The other significant qualitative observation occurred during the cardiovascular stress test. Before the patients walked on the treadmill to take their stress test, the technician explained the entire procedure to them. After a thorough explanation of the procedure, the technician guided the patient slowly through the test. The constant dialogue and support from the technician to the patient helped the patient manage the stress test. Patients who felt heightened anxiety and chest pain were expertly coached by the technician and the physician.

While the physician monitored the printouts from the heart-rate machine and closely observed the patient's progress on the treadmill, the physician also questioned the patient about the precise location and severity of the pain. This questioning provided the physician with further insight into the degree of cardiovascular disorder and also helped to reduce the patient's fears during the stress testing.

Theme Analyses: The Cardiopulmonary Clinic

In my analyses of this fieldwork project, there were two major themes associated with the cardiopulmonary clinic: (1) the compliance rate of patients to scheduled physical examination or interview session; and (2) the miscommunication between health practitioner and patient. According to one of my informants, the rate of noncompliance to scheduled appointments was very high. Approximately, 50% percent of the patients did not make their scheduled appointments. The noncompliance of patients caused technicians and physicians to rearrange constantly their schedules on a regular basis. Since the staff never thoroughly investigated this noncompliance problem, the health practitioners and patients continued to experience difficulties in understanding one another's approach to appropriate health care maintenance.

Perhaps the best example of the miscommunication between the health practitioner and the patient involved the use of the bronchial spray. According to my health practitioner informant in the black lung clinic, patients often misuse the bronchial spray prescribed for their treatment. The major reason for the misuse or nonuse of the bronchial spray is the lack of instruction from the appropriate health practitioner. The informant indicated that this lack of communication and understanding on how to properly use the bronchial spray may be directly related to the poor compliance rate of their patient population. It became apparent again that a lack of understanding on the part of the patients and the health practitioners affected the proper use of the bronchial spray, which is the major immediate treatment procedure for those who are having problems breathing because of the long-term effects of black lung disease.

PHASE 4: REFLECTIVE COMMENTS

In this particular hospital, my ethnographic fieldwork experience provided me firsthand observation of a cardiopulmonary clinic. The primary purpose of this project was to conduct qualitative observations of the relationship between health practitioner and the patient. It soon became apparent, however, that health practitioners and patients experienced varying degrees of miscommunication as it related to the use of the bronchial spray and compliance with scheduled appointments.

Interestingly, at the end of my fieldwork experience, the cardiopulmonary clinic hired a community outreach health worker to address the major problems the clinic had with its patient population. This new employee helped the clinic's staff and health practitioners to better understand and appreciate the social and cultural factors that influence significantly the health-seeking process of the patient population.

Finally, my ethnographic fieldwork project in the Cincinnati hospital helped me to realize the applied role of a medical anthropologist in the clinical setting. The applied medical anthropologist can help the staff to better understand the patient's concepts of culture and health and the relationship of these issues to the outcome of improving patient care.

CONCLUSION

The primary objectives of this applied medical anthropological study were to gain experience in conducting research in a clinical setting and to examine how health care professionals evaluate and treat patients who had experienced environmental health effects such chronic obstructive lung diseases from their occupations.

Surprisingly, there is still relatively little research on environmental health effects on ethnic minority and underserved populations in the United States. The perception is that ethnic minorities and underserved groups are less concerned about their environment than are mainstream middle-and upper-class populations (Brooks et al. 1995). In fact, ethnic minority and underserved groups do not receive adequate representation when confronting environmental occupational problems such as black lung, asthma, or other chronic obstructive lung diseases.

Interestingly, ethnographic methods such as the strategies highlighted in this study were useful in evaluating the treatment procedures of diseases associated with environmental health risks (Benson 1995: 414). Furthermore, ethnographic methods are particularly useful for African Americans primarily because they provide the detailed and insightful investigation of cultural adaptive strategies among African Americans that are often overlooked when treating the African American patient population.

POST-EVALUATION QUESTIONS

1. Describe what type of environmental pollutants are related to black lung disease.

2. Discuss how the cardiopulmonary clinic can implement a broader culturally-sensitive approach to its African American patients.

3. How can the health care professionals better inform African American patients about the proper use of the bronchial spray?

REFERENCES

Benson, Lynette. 1995. "Environmental Health in Minority Communities." In *Environmental Medicine.* Stuart Brooks et al., eds. Pp. 412–415. St. Louis. Mosby..

Brooks, Stuart, M. Gochfeld, R. Jackson, J. Herzstein, and M. Schenker. 1995. *Environmental Medicine.* St. Louis: Mosby.

Cullen, Mark. 1998. "Special Considerations for Developed and Developing Countries." In *International Occupational and Environmental Medicine.* Jessica Herzstein, W. Bunn, L. Fleming, J. Harrington, J. Jeyaratnam, and I. Gardner, eds. Pp. 12–22. St. Louis. Mosby.

Herzstein, Jessica, W. Bunn, L. Fleming, J. Harrington, J. Jeyaratnam, and I. Gardner. 1998. *International Occupational and Environmental Medicine.* St. Louis: Mosby.

Last, John. 1998. *Public Health and Human Ecology.* Stamford, CT: Appleton and Lange.

WEB SITES OF SIGNIFICANCE

Agency for Toxic Substances & Disease Registry: ATSDR

http://atsdr1.atsdr.cdc.gov:8080/atsdrhome.html

National Center for Environmental Health

http://www.cdc.gov/nceh/ncehhome.htm

National Heart, Lung & Blood Institute Asthma Support Organization

http://www.nhlbi.support.com/asthma

National Institute of Environment Health Sciences

http://www.niehs.nih.gov

Chapter 8

Psychosociocultural Stress and African American Women

CRITICAL THINKING QUESTIONS

1. Why is it important to conduct fieldwork at a local public health clinic?

2. Discuss what type of psychosociocultural stressors may affect African American women's health status.

3. How can the applied medical anthropologist help local public clinics to better serve African American women in their community?

INTRODUCTION

Fieldwork in a public health department setting provides the medical anthropologist with a unique opportunity to investigate cultural and health issues of a particular population in that setting. This research project was designed to investigate psychosociocultural stressors of African American mothers and to determine whether there is a relationship between anxiety levels and blood pressure levels. Specifically, the procedure involved analysis of the effects of various environmental factors upon blood pressure, examination of differences or similarities in anxiety among African American mothers, and a test of the validity of the questionnaire on stress. The major quantitative and qualitative findings indicate that psychosociocultural stress is a multifaceted and cultural issue affecting the health status of African American women.

This fieldwork project collected quantitative and qualitative data of African American women who utilized a public health clinic. The fieldwork was conducted from October 1, 1982, to March 22, 1983, at the Cincinnati Health Department's Clement Clinic. The clinic is located approximately six miles from downtown Cincinnati in the predominantly African American community of Avondale.

BACKGROUND INFORMATION

African American women have been portrayed as strong, resilient, and adaptive in their ability to cope with adversity, support their families, and develop avenues of self-esteem and self-actualization (Gibbs and Fuery 1994; Stack 1974). They have been victims of discrimination, economic exploitation, and social rejection for over 370 years (Gibbs and Fuery 1994: 560). Furthermore, they have overcome many of these barriers through developing a set of cultural attitudes, a pattern of coping strategies, and a series of help-seeking behaviors that have enabled them to survive and often thrive in a frequently hostile, exploitive, and unsupportive environment (Gibbs and Fuery 1994).

Despite the new interest in women's health research, very little work has been conducted in the area of African American women's psychosociocultural health issues (Walcott-McQuigg 1996; Hargrove and Keller 1996). Unfortunately, the studies that have been conducted on African American women have been on those in the lower socioeconomic group. The primary aim of this applied medical anthropological fieldwork project was to explore how African American women adapted to the lifestyle stressors of everyday life.

PHASE 1: PREPARING AND ADAPTING TO THE FIELD

To begin this fieldwork project, I wanted to find out which Cincinnati Health Department clinic had the highest African American patient population and which clinic served predominantly the African American community of Avondale. Since I had previously established connections with this community, I was fairly familiar with the surroundings. Although I knew generally the social, cultural, and ethnic dynamics of this community, I was not familiar with the local public health clinics in and around the Avondale community.

In order to get a better understanding of the social, cultural, and ethnic diversity of this community and local public health clinics, I began my observation strategy on October 1, 1983. Once every other week for approximately four months, I spent two to four hours observing five public health clinics in the Cincinnati Public Health district. The Cincinnati Public Health Department had a total of fourteen public health clinics in the metropolitan area.

Each of the five public health clinics that I had decided to observe served a particular patient population. Those who frequented a particular clinic usually were representative of the residents in that community. As the weeks and months passed, I began to get a general idea of the patient population associated with each clinic. By January 1983, I decided that one particular clinic—the Clement Clinic—reflected the type of patient population that I wanted to take part in my study.

This patient population consisted of a diverse (socially, economically, and culturally) sample of African American women. I felt that such a sample would be invaluable in the final analysis of this fieldwork project.

In January, I contacted the administrators of the Cincinnati Health Department with a formal proposal describing my applied medical anthropology fieldwork study. By January 27, I received a reply from the Cincinnati Health Department stating that the Institutional Review Board would like to meet me and to review my project on February 7, 1983. After a thorough, extensive question-and-answer session with the committee, the institutional review board approved my study at the Clement Clinic.

PHASE 2: MEDICAL ANTHROPOLOGY FIELDWORK TECHNIQUES

My participant observation mode began as soon as I completed the review by the internal review board. Once approved by the committee, I was assigned to a head nurse at the Clement Clinic. The head nurse became my key informant to the patient population and all the significant health data that were relevant to my study.

The next phase of my study consisted of conducting semistructured interviews and taking blood pressure measurements of African American female patients using the services of the clinic. The procedure was as follows:

1. The head nurses asked volunteering patients who were waiting in the lobby for their scheduled appointments to take part in my study;
2. In a small office used for the staff lounge, patients were brought to me one by one;
3. After I explained my study to the patients, they signed an informed consent statement;
4. Before I asked any questions, I took the blood pressure of each patient (a Marshal electronic sphygmomanometer and cuff were used to measure blood pressure, and the measurements were periodically checked with a physician for accuracy);
5. Each one-on-one interview lasted approximately fifteen minutes;
6. Anthropometric and environmental variables such as age, weight, height, and soon were all gathered in the interview;
7. I administered a state-trait (stress) anxiety inventory questionnaire (psychosocial stress- evaluating survey) along with medical questions of my own; and
8. I measured blood pressure at the end of the interview.

PHASE 3: ETHNOGRAPHIC FIELDWORK DATA ANALYSES

In phase 3, this applied medical anthropology study primarily focused on the quantitative data collected and analyzed. Of the 71 African American women interviewed, 29 were married, 15 were single parents in relatives' homes, and 27 were single parents living alone. The average age was 30 years, while income ranged from $10,000 to $15,000 per year. Aid to Dependent Children (ADC) contributed 35% of this income. Parental unemployment was 36%, and the average length of unemployment was over one year.

The quantitative data analyses utilized multiple correlations to examine the contributing factors of stress and blood pressure upon the sampled population. The associations between the dependent variables, systolic and diastolic blood pressures, and the demographic and anthropometric variables were examined by multiple regression analyses. To assess potential interaction between anthropometric and environmental variables such as salt, weight, and cigarettes, a simple, stepwise regression (quantitative analyses of each variable's effect on the individual's blood pressure level) was used. Analysis of variance (ANOVA) was utilized in comparisons of state and trait psychosociocultural stress levels and of environmental stressors. A t-test compared the actual differences between single and married women in stress and blood pressure measurements.

Quantitative data analyses revealed three major significant findings. For instance, one of the objectives of this study was to determine the relationship between anxiety and blood pressure. Although there was no significant correlation between blood pressure and scores on the questionnaire, association between weight and number of children with blood pressure was confirmed. Mothers' weight was positively correlated with blood pressure ($r = .48$) whereas number of children in each household was negatively correlated ($r = -.40$). This means that as number of children in the household increase, mothers' blood pressure decreases. Although the direction of this relationship was not expected, it is in accordance with the non-significant correlation between blood pressure and anxiety scores (Bailey 1984: 930).

Another significant quantitative finding was the effect of occupational status. A t test indicated that the mean state anxiety of the unemployed women was 39.4 (SD = 7.1), whereas that for employed women was 34.4 (SD = 7.1; t = 2.7, df = 63, p < .007). For trait anxiety, the pattern was the same (p < .001). Unemployed women's mean trait anxiety was 44.4, while the mean employed women's mean trait score was 36.3.

Interestingly, these particular anxiety scores correlated positively with patients' perceived stress. For instance, patients were asked, "How would you rate your stress level presently on a scale from 1 to 10?" Of the unemployed women 42% rated their perceived stress at 7 or 8, but only 25% of the employed women rated theirs as high (p < .04). In other words, unemployed African American women experienced and expressed higher stress levels than employed African American women.

PHASE 4: REFLECTIVE COMMENTS

Although the sample of African American women was relatively small, the quantitative data substantiate the relationship between psychosociocultural stress and lifestyle. The quantitative data also challenge the belief that African American women do not endure high levels of stress. Depending on their support system and lifestyle, African American women can experience high levels of anxiety that may affect their overall health status.

Interestingly, this study's results found similar results in a number of other studies examining African American women's psychosocial stress issues. Although many questions remain unanswered from all the quantitative data analyses, this study highlighted the importance of psychosociocultural stress upon African American women's mental and physical well-being.

CONCLUSION

Applied medical anthropology fieldwork in a public health setting is challenging and presents the fieldworker with a wide array of unforeseen and uncontrollable health care issues. The major problem that I faced at the clinic was lack of support from my assigned key informants. Although my project was considered to be of value by the Institutional Review Board, some of the clinical staff were not as enthusiastic about the study. Their lack of enthusiasm resulted in the low numbers of patients participating in my study.

For example, the procedure of the study called for me to wait in an office for the nurse to bring volunteering patients. Since some of the nurses thought my research was of no value, patients were not regularly asked to participate. According to clinic procedures, I could not approach the patients myself because my actions may have disrupted patient flow. I therefore waited in the room until my key informant nurse brought volunteering patients to me. Obviously, this procedure hindered not only my ability to get a representative sample but also my ability to ask detailed, in-depth questions of African American women concerning their perceived and actual stress levels.

What are the major implications from this study? First, the psychosociocultural stress inventory can be utilized in a public health setting as an additional tool in diagnosing the effects of stress. Second, we must analyze African American women's needs and their coping strategies to develop socioeconomically and culturally appropriate interventions to reduce their stress, thereby improving their mental and physical well-being.

POST-EVALUATION QUESTIONS

1. What type of additional medical anthropological strategies could I have used in this study?

2. What are the major constraints in conducting a medical anthropological study in a public health clinic?

3. How can health professionals and health care researchers better understand the psychosociocultural stressors of African Americans?

REFERENCES

Bailey, Eric. 1984. "Black Female Parents and Stress." *Psychological Reports* 55: 927–931.

Gibbs, Jewelle and Diana Fuery. 1994. "Mental Health and Well-Being of Black Women: Toward Strategies of Empowerment." *American Journal of Community Psychology* 22: 559–582.

Hargrove, Hazel and Colleen Keller. 1996. "Young Black Women: Defining Health." *Journal of National Black Nurses Association* 3–14.

Stack, Carol. 1974. *All Our Kin: Strategies for Survival in a Black Community.* New York: Harper and Row.

Walcott-McQuigg, Jacqueline and Barbara Logan. 1996. "Preventive Health Practices of African American Women." *Journal of National Black Nurses Association* 49–59.

WEB SITES OF SIGNIFICANCE

National Black Nurses Association

http://www.bronzeville.com/nba/about.html

National Office of Women's Health

http://www.cdc.gov/od/owh/whhome.htm

Western Journal of Black Studies

http://www.wsu.edu:808/~wjbs/archive.htm

Chapter 9

Fieldwork in a Detroit Hospital

CRITICAL THINKING QUESTIONS

1. Why is it important to conduct fieldwork in a hypertension clinic?

2. Discuss the importance of ethnomedical beliefs to patient adherence to prescribed regimen.

3. Describe African Americans pattern of seeking care as it relates to hypertension.

INTRODUCTION

From 1984 to 1988, I was a volunteer in the Hypertension Clinic of Henry Ford Hospital in Detroit. During the first year, I conducted a qualitative study of hypertensive clients. In particular, I became intrigued about the health beliefs and health care utilization patterns among hypertensive clients. After observing staff and client encounters for five months, I realized that a majority of clients had a different perspective than did the professional staff of what constitutes "health" and what constitutes "illness." Moreover, African American clients' perceptions of hypertension and their health-seeking pattern associated with hypertension appeared to be slightly different from those of European American clients. Thus, this qualitative study investigated the issues of the patient's ethnomedical belief system versus the clinician's biomedical belief system. This study also examined alternative health belief systems between African Americans and Euro-American patients.

This fieldwork project used qualitative fieldwork techniques to collect data concerning patients' explanatory models of hypertension. The fieldwork was conducted from May to September 1984 at the Henry Ford Hospital.

BACKGROUND INFORMATION

An explanatory model can be defined as how an individual thinks about health, illness, and disease and how he or she organizes himself/herself toward treatment. Explanatory models can be similar or different from one group to another or one individual to another. Factors that contribute to the similarities or differences of explanatory models are ethnicity, age, sex, socioeconomic grouping, educational level, religiosity, region of the country, and status as new immigrant or native-born.

This qualitative study used hypertension as a means to examine the ethnomedical beliefs and health-seeking pattern of hypertensive patients at a local Detroit hospital primarily because more than 60 million individuals in the United States have elevated blood pressure ($\geq$140/90 mmHg) or have reported being diagnosed by a physician as having hypertension (U.S. Department of Health and Human Services 1986).

Hypertension is the generic term for blood pressure above defined parameters correlated with age. Currently accepted standards defining normal, borderline, and high blood pressure are:

> Normal: up to 138 (systolic) /88 (diastolic)
> Borderline: 140/90 to 158/94
> High: 160/95 and higher

The probable causes of hypertension include heredity, age, sex, stress, excessive weight, high sodium intake, alcohol intake, excessive cigarette smoking, and lack of exercise. Uncontrolled hypertension contributes to death and disability from stroke, coronary disease, and kidney failure (Comprehensive Health Planning Council of Southeastern Michigan 1979).

The prevalence rate of hypertension among African Americans (38.2%) is still substantially higher than among European Americans (28.2%). African Americans, for example, show rates of moderate hypertension that are two times those of European Americans and rates of severe hypertension that are three times greater. This difference in relative frequency is more marked in African American males, among whom the rate of severe elevations (2.2%) is over four times greater than in European Americans (0.5%). Moreover, African American females show the highest prevalence of isolated systolic hypertension (2.4%), which is predominantly seen in the elderly (U.S. Department of Health and Human Services 1985). A disheartening aspect of this health problem in African Americans and other high-risk groups is that adherence to an effective treatment regimen and/or an increased utilization of health screenings can prevent approximately 50% of the deaths associated with hypertension.

The most perplexing attribute of essential hypertension is that there are usually no symptoms associated with it—it is asymptomatic. According to hypertension clinicians, a person cannot tell what his/her blood pressure is by how he or she feels. The only way to know one's pressure is to have it measured.

At the time of measurement, the hypertension clinician should discuss the following items with the patient:

1. the numerical blood pressure value;
2. the need for periodic remeasurement; and
3. available antihypertensive treatment, including specific drugs and results.

In addition, with those individuals whose pressures are elevated, the clinician should inquire about

1. previous treatment for hypertension;
2. the desirability of hypertension control; and
3. the potential dangers of uncontrolled hypertension.

However, most people are unaccustomed to thinking about illness in asymptomatic terms, because symptoms provide the starting point for speculations about illness. Snow (1974) and Blumhagen (1982) contend that individuals develop "commonsense models" or "cultural definitions" of hypertension in an attempt to treat the disease. Such symptoms as headaches, dizziness, tiredness, flushing sensations, and nervousness or anxiety are commonly associated with hypertension. These symptoms, therefore, help to formulate the individual's "cultural definition" or "ethnomedical belief system" of hypertension (Bailey 1991).

PHASE 1: PREPARING AND ADAPTING TO THE FIELD

To begin this fieldwork project, I contacted Henry Ford Hospital's volunteer office and asked if I could volunteer specifically for the Hypertension Clinic. After I met the volunteer director and completed all the forms to become a volunteer, I was asked to return in a week in order for the volunteer office to contact the hypertension clinic and find a place for me to work.

During the week before I reported to the hypertension clinic, I conducted additional background research on hypertension. In particular, I focused upon the problems of adherence to antihypertensive medication among African Americans. Although I had collected a wide array of journal articles stipulating a number of social and behavioral factors contributing to the poor adherence rate among African Americans to antihypertensive regimen, I nonetheless reminded myself to remain as objective as possible when I met patients at the hypertension clinic.

PHASE 2: MEDICAL ANTHROPOLOGY FIELDWORK TECHNIQUES

In this project, the method used was entirely participant observation. The volunteer coordinator informed me that I would actually work in two areas in the hospital: the blood pressure screening program and the hypertension clinic. Each department had two separate functions and two separate identities. My job was to assist primarily with paperwork and sometimes to transport patients to other areas of the hospital.

The blood pressure screening program was close to the entrance of the hospital and staffed entirely by a nurse clinician and an administrative secretary. The blood pressure screening program screened anyone who wanted his or her blood pressure checked. The hypertension clinic, however, was located in an entirely separate building and staffed by renowned physicians, nurse clinicians, technicians, and administrators who served diagnosed hypertensive patients of Henry Ford Hospital.

PHASE 3: ETHNOGRAPHIC FIELDWORK DATA ANALYSES

The following are my first few days of qualitative participant observation at the clinic. These qualitative notes show how I began the process of adapting to the clinical setting.

Day 1: *Today was a very busy and exciting one because this was my first exposure to the blood pressure screening program at Henry Ford Hospital. It is located on the first floor near the entrance. It is important for them to be located here due to the locality for the general public. They have one receptionist and one nurse clinician. Other times, volunteer nurses and clerks help with the screening procedures. The blood pressure screening office is shared with pre-admissions and insurance agency thereby making this area of the hospital fairly crowded. The receptionist explained the procedure to me when they screen a person. There are forms that need to be filled out for the state and the hospital's forms. The receptionist tries to send out a follow-up response to many of the borderline cases as soon as possible. They classify cases into categories such as borderline, high, low, high high and high moderate. Those individuals who are normal on the second screening are not followed-up any further. Yet those who are screened again, and have high blood pressure, they are referred to a physician. Interestingly, the receptionist told me that a few days ago, their office diagnosed a man with a very high reading of blood pressure and then rushed him to the emergency room. He was later admitted to the hospital. What was very interesting about this case was that this man had admitted his mother to the hospital earlier in the day, and later did not feel well. He came to the blood pressure screening office because he experienced signs of dizziness.*

After the first day, my participant observation helped me to begin to understand the culture of the hospital and the health-seeking process of individuals.

Day 2: *Today, I was in the Hypertension clinic and it was really a crazy day. The head nurse was not here and the clinic was basically closed down because most of the doctors were on vacation. Later in the afternoon, I noticed a small degree of friction between the staff. The staff was short-handed so those who were here today had to do extra work. All staff members had to file charts. I was told that this rarely happens but due to the lack of personnel present today, everyone had to assist.*

After the second day, my participant observation helped me to begin to understand the culture of the hypertension clinic.

Day 3: *Today was my first day meeting the nurse clinician in the blood pressure screening clinic. She is the only nurse on staff who does the blood pressure screening. They have two retired nurses who come in and assist and also a volunteer clerk for the receptionist. The procedure for each client is as follows: the client sits down in a chair next to the nurses desk (in a corner). There are pamphlets everywhere in this area informing patients of hypertension. The first couple of questions involve clients' name, address, seen a doctor lately, and any illness. Then the nurse takes the first blood pressure reading. Next, she asks questions about the type of medication the client is taking. If the client cannot remember the name of their medication, the nurse refers to a large book containing all the type of medication for hypertension and all the possible side effects of each medication. After the second reading of the client's blood pressure, the nurse asks some more questions. These questions cover insurance and employment issues. Finally, the third reading of the client's blood pressure is taken. This recording is plotted on the card for the blood pressure screening. The client is given a slip to remind him/her of their blood pressure and their next appointment. The slips are color-coded and indicate whether the client's blood pressure is slightly elevated, moderately elevated, or severely elevated. The nurse informed me that this blood pressure screening program conducts work site visits in areas such as the Fairlane shopping outlet, Chrysler, Sterling Heights, a Latino community center, and a couple of other sites. They find that screening at work sites are very beneficial in getting to the high risk - target population.*

After the third day, my participant observation helped me to better understand the procedure of diagnosing a client with high blood pressure and to realize that the nurse clinician adheres strongly to the *biomedical* approach of hypertension.

Day 12: *Today was a very important day because this was my first time out on a site visit. We went to Fairlane (Dearborn)— the satellite station of Henry Ford Hospital. It's about 15 miles away from the main base of Henry Ford Hospital. This site is an out-patient clinic that caters to the Dearborn community. This site is a new facility with an excellent location near the Fairlane shopping center. Finding the blood pressure screening was no problem. It was located on the 2nd floor in the multi-purpose room. There were 3 volunteers in the afternoon—2 clerical and 1 nurse. Transportation or accessibility to get to the screening was not a problem because there was an elevator for those who had problems with walking.*

One of the first few individuals who wanted their blood pressure checked was a Caucasian women in her late 20s. The first thing that this lady said was, "what are the symptoms of hypertension?" My key informant (nurse clinician) stated that there were none and hypertension is asymptomatic. Interestingly this individual's blood pressure was slightly high and she stated that she has been feeling weird for the past month—"tired & funny." This individual was looking for signs and this weird feeling convinced her to come to this free screening. Additional clients (2, 3, and 5) all claimed that they experienced symptoms with their high blood pressure. Overall, the day was a major success. Yet the actual target population that needs to be aware of their high blood pressure, is not being screened here. Our clients are mainly Fairlane Henry Ford Hospital patients who have a good concept of hypertension and compliance.

Day 16: *In the blood pressure screening clinic, the first client was a Mexican American man in his 40s complaining about symptoms. He stated that he had pain in his chest, numbness on the right side and was having difficulty talking. The nurse clinician informant checked his blood pressure and it was slightly elevated. This client had his blood pressure checked here before several months ago. Today, his blood pressure was definitely elevated. The nurse informant asked me to get a wheelchair in the lobby. The nurse, then, wheeled him to the emergency room. Once she returned from the emergency room, she informed me that this gentlemen appears to have had a mild heart attack. Later, a black male in his 20s had his blood pressure checked. His blood pressure was normal, but he thought his blood pressure was going to be high primarily because he was feeling tired, sick, and uneasy. His spouse accompanied him and she appeared worried.*

PHASE 4: REFLECTIVE COMMENTS

In this participant-observation, qualitative study of hypertension at a Detroit hospital, I learned about the individual's "ethnomedical health belief perception" as it relates to high blood pressure. Interestingly, from a medically orthodox perspective, hypertension is a cardiovascular disease of unknown origin. The most perplexing attribute of hypertension is that there are usually no symptoms associated with it. According to hypertension health professionals, a person cannot tell what his/her blood pressure's by how he/she feels. The only way to know one's pressure is to have it measured.

However, most people are unaccustomed to thinking about high blood pressure in asymptomatic terms because symptoms often provide the starting point for speculations about illness. A majority of the patients who had their blood pressure checked at the blood pressure screening clinic and the hypertension clinic at Henry Ford Hospital felt that they had experienced symptoms associated with their high blood pressure. These symptoms helped to formulate their symptom definition of hypertension.

An individual's symptom definition develops when the degree of discomfort becomes noticeable and acknowledgeable by his or her cultural group. If the illness receives a cultural stamp, then, a health care action follows (Chrisman 1986: 2).

Interestingly, the qualitative findings of this study were quite similar to those Blumhagen's (1982) and Snow's (1976) study of patients at hypertension clinics. In particular, Blumhagen stated the importance of differentiating the explanatory model of hypertension from the health care professional's perspective and the patient's perspective. He stated the following:

At the outset I described the clinical encounter as a set of communications which perhaps should be viewed as a series of transformations: an individual translates unusual sensations into symptoms of illness; the physician translates the symptoms into signs of disease. Unfortunately, the participants are rarely aware that a translation is occurring, or even that multiple languages are being used. This is particularly true when laymen and practitioners refer to the same term in their discourse, not recognizing that the expert use and the lay use of the same word may be far apart. And thus it has proven to be with the terms hypertension and HyperTension. (317)

CONCLUSION

The major objectives of my fieldwork at the hypertension clinic were to become familiar with the clinical aspect of diagnosing and treating hypertension, to get a better understanding of the patient's perspective, and to further develop my skills in applied medical anthropological fieldwork. Fortunately, I accomplished each of these objectives while serving as a volunteer for the hospital.

Interestingly, one outcome that I did not anticipate was my tenure as a volunteer for Henry Ford Hospital. Not only did I serve as volunteer for the period of this project, but I also extended my time as volunteer for four full years of service. Therefore, participant observation has its rewards in service as well as in research.

POST-EVALUATION QUESTIONS

1. How can the day-to-day qualitative fieldwork notes be of benefit to the health care researcher?

2. What are the ethical issues in conducting participant observation in a hospital?

3. How can health care professionals become better informed about the patient's ethnomedical beliefs?

REFERENCES

Bailey, Eric. 1988. "An Ethnomedical Analysis of Hypertension among Detroit Afro-Americans." *Journal of National Medical Association* 80: 1105–1112.

———. 1991. *Urban African American Health Care*. Lanham, MD: University Press of America.

Blumhagen, Dan. 1982. "The Meaning of Hypertension." In *Clinically Applied Anthropology*. Noel Chrisman and Thomas Maretzki, eds. Pp. 297–324. Boston: D. Reidel Publishing Company.

Chrisman, Noel. 1977. "The Health Seeking Process: An Approach to the Natural History of Illness." *Culture and Medical Psychiatry* 1: 351–377.

Comprehensive Health Planning Council of Southeastern Michigan. 1981. Regional Profile 1980. Detroit.

Jones, Paul. 1993. *The Black Health Library Guide to Heart Disease and Hypertension*. New York: Henry Holt.

Snow, Loudell. 1974. "Folk Medical Beliefs and Their Implications for Care of Patients." *Annals of Internal Medicine* 81: 82–96.

———. 1976. "High Blood is Not High Blood Pressure." *Urban Health* 6:54–55.

U.S. Department of Health and Human Services. 1986. *Black and Minority Health: Report of the Secretary's Task Force: IV*. Washington, DC: U.S. Government Printing Office.

WEB SITES OF SIGNIFICANCE

National Heart, Lung & Blood Institute

http://www.nhlbi.nih.gov/nhlbi/nhlbi.htm

Office of Minority Health

http://www.omhrc.gov

Chapter 10

A Needs Assessment of a Prenatal Intervention Program

CRITICAL THINKING QUESTIONS

1. Why is it important to conduct fieldwork in a prenatal health clinic?

2. Describe the most appropriate approach of a medical anthropologist to the problem of prenatal health care.

3. Discuss what type of prenatal care program would be most effective for African American women.

INTRODUCTION

The primary aim of this study was to evaluate the effectiveness of a prenatal health care program in Houston, Texas. The program was named the *Baby Buddy* program and cosponsored by the March of Dimes. We were interested in learning if the program introduced "more" women to prenatal care at an earlier date in their pregnancy and if the program was both appropriate for the educational level of the women and culturally sensitive to their belief system. Qualitative and quantitative data were used to evaluate the prenatal program. Forty-four percent of the sampled mothers began their health care at the clinic during the fourth to sixth month-period of their pregnancy, whereas 41% began during the first to third month-period. Quantitative data analyses showed that expecting mothers' starting prenatal care earlier had a positive effect on the baby's weight ($r = .34$, $p = .02$). In addition to the large percentage of mothers who initially sought health care at the clinic (88%), women often shared the information they learned from the Baby Buddy program (94%). Not only has the program influenced mothers to return to the clinic for preventive health care, but also it has encouraged others to use the clinic services.

This fieldwork project used qualitative and quantitative fieldwork techniques to collect data concerning the effectiveness of the program and the individual mothers who participated in the program. The fieldwork was conducted from March 30, 1989, to December 12, 1989 at the Lyons Avenue Health clinic in Houston.

BACKGROUND INFORMATION

Health care professionals know all too well about the problems of infant mortality and morbidity. Every day, challenging situations arise in the attempt to provide health care for pregnant women or for infants born with problems that could have been prevented.

In 1991, the mortality rate for black infants (17.6) was 2.4 times that for white infants (7.3). Between 1970 and 1991 the mortality rate decreased more for white infants (59%) than for black infants (46%), widening the gap in infant mortality between the two populations. At the heart of the infant mortality rate is the fact that most of the babies' mothers received late or no prenatal care.

Early prenatal care can help (1) decrease infant mortality (death in the first year); (2) prevent low-birth-weight babies (under 5½ pounds), and (3) decrease the cost to taxpayers (approximately low-birth-weight babies may cost up to $1,000 a day in health care) (U.S. Congress 1988).

Despite the growing recognition of the importance of prenatal care as a means of improving birth outcomes, participation rates of pregnant women in prenatal services are relatively low. To counteract such trends, communities throughout the nation are developing and implementing measures to encourage early, regular access to prenatal care. One such program in operation is the Texas Gulf Coast March of Dimes Baby Buddy program.

Nearly one-third of all pregnant women in Houston's health department clinics received late or no prenatal care. In response to that need, the Baby Buddy program began in October 1987. The area selected for the project had a high infant mortality rate (20.5 per 1,000) and a high low-birth-weight rate (10.6 per 1,000).

The primary aim of this study was to evaluate the effectiveness of this new prenatal health care program. The Baby Buddy program is a partnership between the public and private sectors of a community in which people and businesses are recruited to donate time, services, or goods (coupons) to pregnant women receiving health care in a selected clinic. The incentives are donated to pregnant women during their first, second, and third trimesters. Additional coupons are provided during subsequent meetings of the mothers' support group.

The program consists of four variables:

1. public/private support,
2. community education,
3. a mothers' social support group, and
4. clinic participation.

The major goal of this program, therefore, was to develop a community-based approach to increase early and regular prenatal care (Helton 1990).

This Baby Buddy program was located at the Lyons Health Clinic, one of the eleven health clinics serving Houston's metropolitan area. Lyons Health Clinic is bounded to the north by I-10 highway and to the southwest by Magnolia Health Clinic. In 1986, Lyons' population estimate totaled 77,513. African Americans accounted for 65.7% of the population, Anglo-Americans 4.7%, Hispanic/Latin Americans 29.2%, and other 0.4%. Females constituted 51.9% of the population, and males 48.1%. Socioeconomic indicators listed 25.3% of families as under the poverty level and 31.5% of households as headed by single women. The median household income was $12,500 (Wintz 1984).

PHASE 1: PREPARING AND ADAPTING TO THE FIELD

In January 1989, Houston began to increase the public health campaign to address the serious problem of prenatal care in some of the underserved communities in the metropolitan area. Since I had completed a community-based public health project several months prior to this announcement, I was naturally curious about this public health care issue.

To begin this fieldwork project, I contacted the local March of Dimes organization to find out more about the prenatal programs in the city. A few days later, I was referred to an individual working at a prenatal program located at the Lyons Health Clinic. This individual, a nurse-clinician and innovator of this Baby Buddy program, became my key informant. Once I contacted and introduced myself to my key informant, she invited me to attend a prenatal session at the clinic.

PHASE 2: MEDICAL ANTHROPOLOGY FIELDWORK TECHNIQUES

Overall, this project consisted of three stages: (1) qualitative observation and participant observation of prenatal Baby Buddy sessions for mothers and family members; (2) preparing a draft proposal to conduct an evaluation of the program; and (3) conducting quantitative analyses of a semistructured questionnaire evaluating the effectiveness of the program.

On March 30, 1989, I began my observations and participant observations of Baby Buddy mothers' group session. The group was a forum where many special issues were discussed. Mothers shared information and comments with facilitators on topics such as the process of birth, and sex, social, economic, and cultural issues. I attended a total of four Baby Buddy Mothers' group sessions from March 30 to May 4, 1989.

From the end of May to August, I worked on a proposal to present to the March of Dimes. The research proposal major objectives were to determine if the program would introduce more women to prenatal care at an earlier date in their pregnancy and if the program would be both appropriate for the educational level of the women and culturally sensitive to their belief system. I therefore designed a semistructured questionnaire to collect the data. By the end of September, my proposal was well received by the local administrators of the March of Dimes. By October, I received official approval to conduct the evaluation.

Stage 3 of this project began soon after the official approval. In cooperation with the March of Dimes Baby Buddy program, the research team (a community health nurse "key informant," an independent volunteer and I) conducted a three-month study to determine the effectiveness of this program for mothers. A random sample of 32 mothers constituted the study's sample. Potential subjects were contacted by the independent volunteer and asked to participate via the telephone. The projected sample of 50 mothers was reduced due to the difficulties of locating former Baby Buddy mothers and the fact that this program was relatively brand new. All interviews were conducted by phone, lasting approximately 45–60 minutes.

Data from the semistructured questionnaire were coded and entered onto the computer at the University of Houston using the Statistical Package for Social Sciences (SPSS). The data analyses sought to access the factors related to perceptions of pregnancy, delivery, child-raising and health care seeking. Standard parametric statistics tested the Baby Buddy indices and sociodemographic variables associated with the participants.

PHASE 3: ETHNOGRAPHIC FIELDWORK DATA ANALYSES

Qualitative Analyses: The Prenatal Program

During my first qualitative observation of the Baby Buddy program, I observed a total of six pregnant mothers (three African American and three Hispanic American) sharing their thoughts and asking questions with the facilitator (my key informant) of the mothers' group. After my key informant introduced me, I moved to the back of the room to observe the interactions. Although I thought my presence would make a difference in the group's conversation, it was apparent within a couple of minutes that the mothers and the facilitator were not apprehensive in sharing the most intimate details in this setting.

During the one-and-a-half hour session, my key informant and the mothers dialogued so well and talked about so many topics that it was hard to imagine that this group had started only a couple of weeks prior to my visit. Basically, the facilitator and the mothers covered four major topics:

1.   The role of the Baby Buddy program to the mother;
2.   Sexual activity and protection from sexually transmitted diseases;
3.   Effects of drug use on the baby; and
4.   Cultural beliefs concerning pregnancy.

In particular, cultural beliefs concerning pregnancy became a major issue for many of the young mothers. The following are examples of beliefs about pregnancy:

1.   If you eat spicy foods, it will burn the baby's eyes.
2.   Mothers sleep pattern will affect baby's sleep pattern.
3.   If you sit a certain way, the umbilical cord will strangle the baby.
4.   If certain people touch you or look at you (evil eye), they can give the baby bad spirits.
5.   If the mother looks at frightening objects or things, the baby will be easily frightened.
6.   If mothers have intercourse while pregnant, it will affect the baby.

By the end of the session, the facilitator appeared to have not only dispelled a number of misconceptions of pregnancy but also helped the mothers to gain confidence in themselves and their babies' health.

When I returned for sessions 2, 3, and 4, my role as strictly an observer changed to a participant observer. My key informant and the mothers encouraged my participation in the group's activities. In fact, during session 3, in which there were twenty women and two men, including myself, I was asked to participate in a childbirth role-playing exercise. After all of us reviewed a film on childbirth, the facilitator asked the group to practice childbirth role playing. I therefore was paired with one of the young mothers.

The goal of the childbirth role-playing exercise was to emphasize three major objectives for mothers and their childbirth partner: (1) confidence, (2) relaxation, and (3) breathing pattern. The facilitator shared with us that during childbirth it is important for the mother and the childbirth partner to maintain their confidence, continue to find ways to relax, and maintain a steady and even breathing pattern.

Yet not only was my participant observation in this particular activity to know what happens to expecting mothers during childbirth, but my participation enlightened me on how effective this Baby Buddy mothers' support group was to those who participated. The mothers in this group "bonded" and found a positive environment/setting in which they received encouragement and support for their pregnancy. If I had not participated in the group's activities, I may not have truly understood the cultural and psychological impact of this program to the mothers. Additionally, the qualitative observations and participant observations helped me to develop a preliminary proposal to conduct an evaluation of the effectiveness of this program for the mothers.

Quantitative Analyses: The Prenatal Program and Maternal Child Issues

The data analyses sought to determine at what stage a mother began prenatal care, sociocultural factors related to perceptions of pregnancy, child-raising issues, and the health care-seeking pattern of mothers. The significant maternal child care findings were as follows:

1. Forty-five percent of the sample mothers began their health care at the clinic during the fourth to sixth-month period of their pregnancy, whereas 41% began during the first-to third-month period.
2. A majority of women (86%) used the Lamaze technique learned in the Baby Buddy program.
3. Only 6% of the mothers' babies experienced health problems.
4. A majority of mothers returned to the clinic for such services as individual checkup (75%), well baby checkup (78%), baby immunization (69%), and family planning (66%).

Perhaps the most significant findings concerning maternal child care issues involved the relationship between the baby's weight and two important sociocultural issues—educational level of the mother and the time when the mother began prenatal health care. A Pearson correlation showed that expecting mother's starting prenatal care earlier had a positive effect on the baby's weight. That is, as mothers started prenatal care earlier, the baby's weight tended to show a positive increase ($r = .34$, $p = .02$).

In addition, further statistical analyses revealed a relationship between the baby's weight and the educational level of the mother. As the mother's educational level increased, it had a positive biological impact on the baby's weight ($r = .37$, $p = .02$). In fact, babies tended to be heavier for mothers who had a higher educational level. Thus, two significant sociocultural factors related to the baby's weight at birth: (1) the educational level of the mother and (2) the time when mothers began prenatal care at the Lyons Clinic.

Quantitative Analyses: The Baby Buddy Program

Another major focus of the data analyses helped to assess the impact of the Baby Buddy program on the lives of the mothers. The major findings of the Baby Buddy program issues were as follows ($p = .05$):

1. One hundred percent of the mothers agreed that the Baby Buddy mothers' program had helped them.
2. Eighty-one percent of the mothers strongly agreed that the staff really seemed to care about them and their baby's health.
3. Seventy-eight percent of the mothers strongly agreed that the staff explained things in words they could understand.

4. Seventy-one percent of the mothers strongly agreed that the staff let them tell the staff what they thought was important.
5. Ninety-four percent of the mothers shared the information learned from the Baby Buddy program with others.
6. Ninety-one percent of the mothers have brought other pregnant women to the clinic or encouraged pregnant women to get health care.
7. Sixty-six percent of the mothers stated that they have achieved or started on their goals.
8. Eighty-four percent of the mothers indicated that the coupons and gifts encouraged them to return.
9. Ninety-four percent of the mothers indicated that they have told others about the gifts/coupons.

A hierarchical multiple regression assessed which factors contributed the most variance to the number of sessions attended at the Lyons clinic by mothers. Of all the sociodemographic variables in question, six major factors contributed 60% of the variance. Of these, employment (B =.40), residence pattern (B =.48), age (B =.60), currently in school (B- =.60), total family income (B =.27), and educational level (B =.25) were statistically significant (p = .05). In other words, those women who were employed, lived with close relatives, were older, were currently in school, had a moderate income level, and had a higher educational level attended more sessions at the clinic. Thus, these sociodemographic factors played an important role in the participation of mothers in the Baby Buddy program.

Qualitative Analyses: The Baby Buddy Program

One of the major objectives of this evaluation was to assess the qualitative impact of the Baby Buddy program on the women who participated in the program. The following comments are typical responses to the question, Have you achieved or started on any of the goals you talked about in the Baby Buddy group?

"Getting my GED (general equivalency diploma) and working on
   computers."
"Finishing school."
"Raising my son and finishing high school."
"Being a good mother and work."
"Losing weight."
"A positive frame of mind."

Perhaps the most touching response came from a mother who simply stated, *"The Baby Buddy program got my family back on line."* The positive psychosocial impact of this program on the well-being of mothers was quite evident quantitatively and qualitatively.

If there were any suggestions offered by women to improve the Baby Buddy program, they focused upon possibly expanding the services of the program. Women responded as follows:

"Include classes for fathers."

"Women need play pens and walkers for children."

"More classes about teen pregnancy, sexual diseases, low birthright babies and drugs."

"Classes on another day."

Although the Baby Buddy program was a group-oriented counseling service, a few women preferred individual counseling. The following comment stressed this particular issue: *"I need individual counseling because I may not want to talk about my pregnancy with the group."* Whether to include more group classes or individualized counseling, the qualitative findings from the semi-structured questionnaire supported the positive impact of the Baby Buddy program on the lives of the women.

Quantitative Analyses: Health Care Seeking Pattern of Pregnant Teenage Women

Health care seeking is a series of steps taken by a woman who perceives a need for help as she attempts to adapt to the various stages of pregnancy. The findings were as follows:

1. A majority of the mothers were proud (47%) when they learned of their pregnancy.
2. A majority of the mothers (53%) indicated that one's significant other was the first person they told about their pregnancy. Interestingly, younger mothers (fifteen to nineteen years) told their significant other (64%) and others (29%) as opposed to their mothers (0%) or no one else (7%).
3. A vast majority of the mothers (88%) initially sought health care at the clinic.
4. Mothers indicated that some of their friends (34%) were not aware of the services or do not visit doctors/nurses for health problems.
5. A majority of the mothers (81%) feel that they did not have any transportation problems.
6. Approximately 31% of the mothers attended the Baby Buddy's group sessions a total of five to ten sessions.

In addition to the large percentage of mothers who initially sought health care at the clinic (88%), mothers often shared the information they learned from the Baby Buddy program with friends (94%).

Qualitative Analyses: Health Care Seeking Pattern of Teenage Mothers

Personal, qualitative accounts such as the following typify *how* and *why* mothers shared information with their network about the Baby Buddy program:

> "I told my sister and two friends— Lamaze and Baby Buddy
>   helped a lot."
> "Baby Buddy helps you when you get scared."
> "Baby Buddy helps us to dispel some of the old wives' tales
>   of pregnancy."

Perhaps the most interesting response about the Baby Buddy program was as follows: *"Before I told my friend that the Baby Buddy program makes you feel good, she felt that it was the end of the world and she couldn't survive."* It was quite apparent that word of mouth or one's lay network and referral network helped significantly to promote the social and health care services associated with the Baby Buddy program.

PHASE 4: REFLECTIVE COMMENTS

The qualitative and quantitative findings of this study helped to highlight the positive impact that mothers received from participating in the Baby Buddy program. Not only has the program influenced mothers to return to the clinic for prenatal care, but it has also encouraged others to join the Baby Buddy mothers' support group.

There were four major reasons for the success of the support group. First, the group was open; no appointment was necessary. The weekly meeting was set on a busy clinic day, and women were allowed to come and go as their schedules required. They were encouraged to bring other women, significant others, support persons, and children as desired.

Second, the group was issue-oriented, and usually the mothers set the agenda. Sometimes one issue was raised, and it alone was discussed. Issues ranged from pregnancy changes, to neighborhood drug problems, to family violence, to employment and education.

Third, time was allocated during each meeting to present core information about labor and delivery, pregnancy, and parenting. At least once a month, a Baby Buddy instructor from the private sector was scheduled to present an educational program.

Finally, the meetings were a time for sharing. Mothers were encouraged to share telephone numbers with each other and to share the knowledge of the Baby Buddy program with friends in the community. Included in their responsibility of participating in the program, they participated in a seminar and tour of a neonatal intensive care unit at a local hospital. After the seminar and tour, the mothers were given certificates that designated them as Baby Buddy resource mothers. Thus, all mothers who participated in the program shared this information with their community.

CONCLUSION

The findings of this applied medical anthropology project indicated that the Baby Buddy program made a significant impact on the well-being of these mothers and their babies. Moreover, this study reaffirmed previous studies concerning the importance of early prenatal care on mothers and their babies. Expectant mothers who started prenatal care earlier tended to have healthier babies. Therefore, comprehensive prenatal care programs that work closely within the psychosociocultural orientation of the mother will exhibit better success rates than those prenatal programs that do not.

Finally, our evaluation of this Baby Buddy program convinced local public health agencies in Houston to expand this social support and case-finding activity from one clinic to six clinics in the metropolitan area. As a result, thousands of pregnant women benefited from participating in the Baby Buddy prenatal program.

POST-EVALUATION QUESTIONS

1. Describe the applied medical anthropological strategies used in this study.

2. Discuss how you would have improved this study.

3. Describe how sociocultural factors played a significant role with African American women and prenatal care.

REFERENCES

Helton, Anne. 1990. "A Buddy System to Improve Prenatal Care." *American Journal of Maternal/Child Nursing* 15: 234–237.

U.S. Congress, Office of Technology Assessment. 1988. *Healthy Children: Investing in the Future*. Washington DC: U.S. Government Printing Office.

Wintz, C. 1984. "Blacks." In *the Ethnic Groups of Houston*, ed. F. Mehdan. Pp. 9–40. Houston: Rice University Studies.

WEB SITES OF SIGNIFICANCE

Centers for Disease Control and Prevention: Office of Women's Health: Reproductive Health

http://www.cdc.gov/od/owh/whrh.htm

March of Dimes

http://www.modimes.org

National Institute of Child Health & Human Development

http://www.nih.gov/nichd

Chapter 11

Culturally Competent Health Screening Programs

CRITICAL THINKING QUESTIONS

1. Why is it important to conduct fieldwork in a community health clinic?

2. Describe the approach of the medical anthropologist in reaching the local African American community.

3. Discuss the strategy of the medical anthropologist in working with the local public health officials.

INTRODUCTION

Community health screening programs were originally designed to stimulate change in family and community knowledge and behavior relating to the prevention of disease; to inform about the use of available health resources; and to improve the environmental, economic, and educational factors related to health. Since their inception, however, community health screening programs have primarily used conventional approaches to health improvement for the African American community. That is, the need is not merely for the provision of more preventive and curative health services or the distribution of services to passive recipients but for the active involvement of local populations in ways that will preserve or repattern their knowledge, attitudes and motivation concerning major health care issues. Health care professionals such as clinicians need to expand their biopsychosocial model to include specific sociocultural data concerning African American health care-seeking patterns. Collaborative efforts of this type therefore enable health care professionals to design future community health screening programs for the African American community that are practical and culturally competent.

This fieldwork project used qualitative fieldwork techniques to collect data on a local community health clinic and the population it served in order to develop a culturally competent health screening project. The fieldwork was conducted from October 20, 1988, to April 22, 1989, at the Riverside Health Clinic in Houston, Texas.[1]

BACKGROUND INFORMATION

Community health screening programs were originally designed (1) to stimulate change in family and community knowledge and behavior relating to the prevention of disease; (2) to inform the use of available health resources; and (3) to improve the environmental, economic, and educational factors related to health (Geiger 1972). Since their inception during the 1960s and 1970s, however, community health screening programs have primarily used conventional approaches to health improvement. That is, the need is not merely for the prevention and curative health services to passive recipients, but for the active involvement of local populations in ways which will preserve or repattern their knowledge, attitudes and motivation concerning major health care issues.

With regard to community health screening programs being "culturally-competent," this term refers to another level of public health intervention. Cultural competence has three components: purpose, attitude, and skills. The purpose of cultural competence is to achieve improved health outcomes. Attitude is the willingness to adapt oneself to others' needs. Skills are those competencies or behaviors that exemplify correctness of technique in interactions between the professional and the patient. Thus, when health care professionals design a culturally competent community health screening program, it is intended to address five major issues:

1. to alert a target group to health issues,
2. to help them make choices,
3. to maintain some of their traditional health care practices,
4. to encourage them to try new health care practices, and
5. to inform them of the most straightforward and effective behavioral alternatives for health promotion.

Population

From the early 1970s to the 1980s, Houston established itself as the premier city in the sunbelt. The prominence of the city was highlighted by such characteristics as being one of the fastest growing cities in the nation (from 1.74 million in 1970 to 2.4 million in 1980), leading the nation in home construction (over 487,000 housing units were added to the area in the 1970s), and serving as a magnet attracting individuals seeking expanding opportunities (U.S. Bureau of Census 1982).

African American Population

While Houston's African American population continues to expand outward to all five wards of the city, the largest African American enclaves are in the Fourth Ward, southwest of downtown around the old Freedmantown neighborhood; in the Third Ward, southeast of downtown; and in the Fifth Ward, northeast of the business district (Wintz 1984). The Third Ward serves as the hub of African American social, cultural, and economic life in Houston. The Third Ward also serves as a center of African American higher education, with the nation's third largest historically African American university, Texas Southern University. African American mass communications, with three leading African American Houston newspapers and the three African American-owned radio stations, and African American cultural, civil rights, and political awareness organizations' headquarters are also located in the Third Ward (Bullard 1982).

One of the problems that confronted Houston's African American population was a substandard health care system. The African American health care system that developed during the period of segregation has all but disappeared. Of the four African American hospitals still operating in the city in 1970, only two, Riverside General Hospital in the Third Ward and Charles Drew Hospital, were still open in 1989. In an effort to relieve the problems of available health care to African Americans and other ethnic populations, the city of Houston's Department of Health and Human Services expanded its operations of health clinics in the Houston area.

In 1986, Riverside's population estimate totaled 69,798. Blacks accounted for 77.5% of the population, whites for 12.9%, Hispanics for 7.5% of the population, and Others for 2.1%. Males constituted 48.2% of the population, and females 51.8%.

The average age of the overall population fell within the 25–29 year group. The average age of Hispanics and others was within the 20–24 year group. Blacks' had an average within the 25–29 year-age group and Whites had an average age within the 30–34 year-age group.

Socioeconomic indicators listed 24.0% of families as under the poverty level and 36.1% of households as headed by single females. The median household income for 1989 was $17,500.

PHASE 1: PREPARING AND ADAPTING TO THE FIELD

After I completed a cultural-historical and sociodemographic library research on the Riverside residential area, I volunteered to serve on the Community Advisory Board of Riverside Health Clinic. On January 20, 1988, I became a member of the Community Advisory Board. Riverside's Community Advisory Board mainly consisted of local Third Ward residents, Houston Health Department officials, and local business people. The functions of the Advisory Board entailed overseeing the operations of the clinic and developing community programs. Board meetings were held once a month at Riverside Health Clinic.

To find out more about Riverside's African American community, I established a working dialogue and association with three key informants in this area: Shannon Jones (Riverside medical director), a physician (Riverside medical director), and Mrs. Helen Hall Kinard (president of the Advisory Board for the Riverside Health Center). These three informants were instrumental not only in the conceptualization and implementation of the community health screening but also in providing substantive qualitative data about Houston Health Department's program procedures and Third Ward residents' needs.

PHASE 2: MEDICAL ANTHROPOLOGY FIELDWORK TECHNIQUES

Overall, the procedure of this medical anthropological fieldwork project involved four major stages: (1) library research of Houston's African American communities, particularly the Riverside residential area; (2) participant observation as member of the Community Advisory Board; (3) informal interviews of residents in the Third Ward area; and (4) advocate as chairperson of the community health fair.

Once the 1989 spring agenda was established, I was elected chairperson of the 1989 Riverside Health Fair by the Advisory Board. My job was to organize, coordinate, and direct all the operations of the health fair. To get to know more of the personal and health care dynamics of local community residents, I spent as many hours as I could at the Riverside Health Clinic.

I conducted qualitative interviews of personnel associated with the clinic, nearby neighbors, and professionals in the community. In particular, I interviewed a key administrative informant, Ernest Gibson, from the historical black hospital, Riverside General Hospital. The qualitative data that I gathered from this key administrative person as well as from individuals from all walks of life enabled me to arrive at a conclusion on the overall design of this upcoming health fair.

PHASE 3: ETHNOGRAPHIC FIELDWORK DATA ANALYSES

Qualitative Analyses: Designing the Culturally Competent Health Fair

The qualitative information I gathered from those who worked at the clinic and from those who lived in the neighborhood suggested that for the average household the priority placed on maintaining "health" had to be adjusted in light of economic and social needs. I concluded that since unemployment and public safety were major issues affecting most community residents, residents needed information on job opportunities and public safety strategies for the young and elderly as much as they needed traditional health messages.

As chairperson of the health fair, I therefore proposed a modification to the original design of the health fair, primarily because the model was outdated and not oriented to the local African American community. The proposed change— to holistically address the sociocultural parameters of community health— stimulated much controversy.

Initially, board members considered that a typical health fair should offer strictly medical services to local residents. Medical services such as cholesterol screening, blood pressure screening, vision screening, and height/weight assessment were the traditional norm for a public health fair. Yet after much debate among Advisory Board members and support of two key informants (president of the Advisory Board and health center administrator), the health fair was finally expanded to include a wide array of health care and social services in an effort to meet the needs of Third Ward residents, that is, designing a health fair as a community festival instead of the typical annual health fair. Designing the health fair as a community festival and selection of the alternative type of services were based on three criteria:

1. Do the services address current problems in the community?;
2. Do the services require residents to rely upon African American institutions in the community?; and
3. Do the services help people discover ways to reduce the fear about health and seek health care in the community?

In cooperation with Houston's Department of Health and Human Services and eighteen local agencies, basic tests and preventive health services offered at the Riverside community health fair: height and weight screening, dental screening, pulmonary function screening, prenatal and child care counseling, law enforcement child identification screening, social service counseling, and AIDS counseling and an AIDS education play. In addition, this daylong, free community health screening provided food and prizes to all participants. The idea was that learning about how to keep the community healthy should be a festive occasion organized in celebration of African American community life.

Qualitative Analyses: Operating the Culturally Competent Health Fair

After five months of planning, organizing, and soliciting support from local African American health care and social agencies, Riverside's 1989 health fair proved a major success. An initial projection was for 70 participants. Well over 200 local residents of all age groups participated. Approximately 90% of the participants were African American, 5% Euro-Americans and 5% Hispanic/Latino American. The proportion of African American participants was even higher than their proportion in the local population. The decision to concentrate on the local African American population was primarily because of the low numbers of African Americans who actually used the clinic as their source of health care.

Although I was busy managing the community health screening, I noticed that most individuals arrived with several extended family members belonging to either a young age group (approximately 3–16 years) or a mature age group (approximately 50–80 years). It was obvious that individuals who sought health care/social services did so as groups of family or household groupings. In addition, the health fair was perceived not only as a "health fair" but as a "community event" and it promoted community trust in local health professionals. Thus, the intention that the advisory committee organizers of Riverside's health fair had of reaching out to local residents proved a fruitful endeavor for the entire community.

PHASE 4: REFLECTIVE COMMENTS

The major objective of the health fair was to provide health care and social services for an African American community in a culturally competent and practical approach. The culturally competent approach consisted of:

1. increasing the number of African American health care and social service personnel who could participate in the fair;
2. promoting the event through traditional African American media; and
3. educating African Americans in a style and pattern that they could understand and were accustomed to.

For example, all agencies were encouraged strongly to have a diversified staff work their booth. This strategy helped many of the participants feel more comfortable asking questions and helped them develop an immediate rapport with the agency's workers. The Advisory Board also enlisted the services of the local African American radio station not only to announce the health fair but also to bring their special mobile van to play music. In addition, we advertised the health fair in the local, well-established African American newspaper.

Moreover, the AIDS educational play provided an example of how to educate and discuss serious health issues in an entertaining and culturally sensitive approach. The playwright was an African American male, and the performers were young adults. Thus, the play had dialogue and issues directly reflecting young African American lifestyles. Because of excellent rapport that the African American playwright and the community theater group had already established with Houston's African American population, the AIDS play worked well.

Community health screening programs must emerge from a knowledge of, and a respect for, the culture of the target community to ensure that both the community organization and development effort and any interventions that emerge are culturally competent and linguistically appropriate.

CONCLUSION

This fieldwork project demonstrated how applied medical anthropologists are capable of fathoming the needs and peculiarities of major health care issues. The culturally competent intervention strategies developed for the Houston community can be best summarized as:

1. involving individuals/group members in the planning process to maximize the likelihood that they will have an investment in the outcomes;
2. combining knowledge of sociocultural and psychosocial factors to produce the most favorable outcomes by targeting specific and known community needs and by not isolating physical health from overall community wellness;
3. using anthropological concepts and data to inform organizers more comprehensively about the cultural context, emphasizing aspects of which they had previously been unaware.

POST-EVALUATION QUESTIONS

1. How could have this project been improved?

2. Why are culturally competent health screening programs more effective than generic health screening programs?

3. How can public health administrators develop health screening programs more culturally competent?

ENDNOTE

1. Portions previously published in *Practicing Anthropology* (Winter 1994, Volume 16, Number 4), "Medical Anthropologist as Health Department Consultant."

REFERENCES

Bailey, Eric. 1994. "The Medical Anthropologist as Health Department Consultant." *Practicing Anthropology* 16: 13–15.

Bullard, R. 1982. *Houston's Third Ward: A Center of Black Business*. Houston: Texas Southern University Press.

Geiger, H. 1972. "A Health Center in Mississippi: A Case Study in Social Medicine." In *Medicine in a Changing Society*. L. Corey, S. Saltman, and M. Epstein, eds. St. Louis: C.V. Mosby.

U.S. Bureau of Census. 1982. *Provisional Estimates of Social and Economic and Housing Characteristics*. Washington, DC: U.S. Government Printing Office.

Wintz, C. 1984. "Blacks." In *The Ethnic Groups of Houston*. F. Mehdan ed. Pp. 9–40. Houston, TX: Rice University Studies.

WEB SITES OF SIGNIFICANCE

Department of Health & Human Services

http://www.os.dhhs

Healthy People 2000

http://odphp.osophs.dhhs.gov/pubs/hp2000/

Chapter 12

The Diabetic Patient's Adaptation to Outpatient Clinic

CRITICAL THINKING QUESTIONS

1. Why is it important to conduct fieldwork in a diabetes clinic?

2. Discuss the major reasons African Americans experienced difficulty in adhering to the diabetic regimen.

3. Describe how the applied medical anthropologist contributed to the understanding of the diabetes patient.

INTRODUCTION

As a population, African Americans are at increased risk for developing diabetes mellitus. African Americans also experience higher rates of at least three of the serious complications of diabetes: blindness, amputations, and end-stage renal disease. The primary objective of this study was to assess the relationship between health beliefs and patterns of health service utilization in two populations with non-insulin dependent diabetes that are economically similar but culturally distinctive: African Americans and Euro-Americans. In cooperation with the Regenstrief Health Center at Indiana University, the research team conducted a two-year qualitative and quantitative study to examine the health beliefs and health care-seeking pattern of African Americans and Euro-American diabetic patients. Qualitative findings were as follows: (1) assess the patient's cause of the diabetes; (2) attempt to address any misconception of diabetes; and (3) adjust the diabetic regimen to the individual's social and ethnic lifestyle pattern.

This fieldwork project used qualitative and quantitative data collection techniques to investigate health beliefs and health care-seeking pattern of African American and Euro-American diabetics. The fieldwork project was conducted in two phases at the diabetes clinic in the Regenstrief Health Center at Indiana University, Indianapolis. The two phases consisted of (1) qualitative phase 1: June–August 1991; and (2) qualitative and quantitative phase 2: June–December 1992.

BACKGROUND INFORMATION

Diabetes is a chronic disease of pancreatic origin, characterized by insulin deficiency. There are two main types of diabetes, caused by different problems. In type I diabetes, the body makes little or no insulin; whereas in type II, the body makes insulin but cannot use it.

Insulin-dependent diabetes (type I) affects approximately one in ten people with diabetes. Although it begins most often when people are young, it may also occur in older adults. Research indicates that the major factors related to type I diabetes are (1) a history of type I diabetes in the family; (2) viruses that have injured the pancreas; and (3) a problem with the body's defense system that had destroyed the insulin-making cells in the pancreas. The symptoms include increased thirst, increased passing of urine, increased hunger, sudden weight loss, and feeling very tired (U.S. DHHS 1990; Harris 1987).

Non-insulin dependent diabetes (type II) is the most common form of diabetes. Approximately nine out of ten people with diabetes have type II. Although it can occur in younger people, it most often begins when people are over 40 years of age (U.S. DHHS 1990; Harris 1987).

The symptoms of type II include feeling tired, dryness, itchy skin, frequent infections, frequent passing of urine, blurred eyesight, numbness or tingling in hands or feet, increased hunger, and increased thirst. The exact cause of type II is unknown, but it tends to occur in people who are (1) 40 years old or older, (2) overweight, (3) African American, (4) Hispanic/Latino American, and (5) Native American and those who have (1) a family history of diabetes; (2) had diabetes during a pregnancy; (3) stress of an illness or injury; and (4) high blood pressure.

As a population, African Americans are at increased risk for developing diabetes mellitus. The age-adjusted prevalence of non-insulin-dependent diabetes among African Americans is 91% higher than in non-Hispanic whites, with the number of diagnosed cases increasing fourfold in just over two decades from 228,000 in 1963 to approximately 1 million in 1985 (U.S. DHHS 1990). This is almost double the rate of increase among white, non-Hispanic Americans.

As many as 15% of African American women, aged 20–30 years have impaired glucose tolerance, and the incidence of diabetes is at least twice as great in African Americans aged 35–55 years than in whites (Harris 1990; Drury et al. 1985; and Otten et al. 1990).

African Americans' increased risk of diabetes is independent of all major sociodemographic factors such as age, sex, educational level, marital status, living arrangement, and regional category. However, diabetes is more prevalent among African Americans living in the central city and those living in the western United States (Ruderman et al. 1990; Gohdes 1988; Glascow and Toobert 1988).

In 1987, diabetes and its complications were the seventh leading cause of death in Indiana and the sixth leading cause of death among African Americans in Indiana (Interagency State Council on Black and Minority Health 1992). From 1980 to 1986, the diabetes rates in Indiana exceeded U.S. rates. Between 1982 and 1986, African American males and females had the highest age-adjusted death rates, respectively in Indiana from diabetes.

PHASE 1: PREPARING AND ADAPTING TO THE FIELD

In 1991, I was contacted by the Indiana University Diabetes Research and Training Center to assist a team of researchers who wanted to investigate the role that culturally influenced health beliefs play in both disease status and health service utilization of African Americans with non-insulin-dependent diabetes (NIDDM) or type II diabetes mellitus. Once I met with the project director (physician) and the team of behavioral scientists in the School of Medicine, I felt that I could contribute substantially to the intervention phase of this study.

My specific goals were (1) to develop and to validate a health belief assessment tool that is responsive to the cultural perspectives of African Americans and (2) to administer the health belief assessment tool to two NIDDM patient samples and determine the relationship between the patients' beliefs and actual usage of health care services. It was expected that the health belief assessment tool would be incorporated into the data collection for the larger-scale study under way and that the instrument could assist in predicting adherence with the diabetes regimens in this population.

PHASE 2: MEDICAL ANTHROPOLOGY FIELDWORK TECHNIQUES

In order to accomplish the specific goals, I designed a three-phase approach to my study: (1) conduct a five-month qualitative study of patients attending the diabetic clinic (June 1, 1991–October 31, 1991); (2) conduct a three-   month qualitative and quantitative study of African American and Euro-American patients attending the diabetic clinic (June 1, 1992–August 31, 1992); (3) test and analyze a quantitative and qualitative culturally sensitive assessment tool.

During phase 1, in cooperation with the Regenstrief Health Center and the Diabetes Research and Training Center, I conducted a five-month study of patients attending the Diabetic Clinic. Qualitative observations and informal interviews were gathered from physicians, nurses, staff members, and patients in an attempt not only to comprehensively understand the sociocultural dynamics of the diabetic patient but also to prepare the principal investigator for conducting a clinically applied anthropological study.

The diabetes patient population was selected from the diabetes population treated at the Wishard Memorial Hospital located on the Indiana University Medical School campus (Regenstrief Health Center). Wishard Memorial Hospital is a 540-bed general medical/surgical hospital that primarily serves the inner-city residents of Indianapolis. It is owned by the county Health and Hospital Corporation and is operated by the Indiana University School of Medicine.

All physicians practicing at Wishard Memorial Hospital are either faculty or house staff of Indiana University School of Medicine. There are more than 20,000 admissions to the inpatient service each year, approximately 5,000 of whom are admitted to the medical service.

Phase 2 consisted of qualitative observations, informal interviews, and semistructured interviews of patients in the Diabetes Clinic. The primary purpose of phase 2 was to determine patients' perceptions of the cause of the diabetic condition and symptoms and common side effects of their diabetic treatment regimen. Interviews were conducted with subjects in an outpatient clinic setting after they completed their scheduled clinic appointment.

The semistructured questionnaire was used to assess the health beliefs and health care- seeking pattern of the diabetic patient. Items that significantly predicted variance were utilized in construction of the African American Health Belief Inventory (AAHBI ©). The AAHBI was based upon on subjects' responses to the following instruments:

1.   Health Belief Model;
2.   Diabetes Symptom Questionnaire;
3.   medical care satisfaction; and
4.   a structured clinical interview.

PHASE 3: ETHNOGRAPHIC FIELDWORK DATA ANALYSES

Phase 3 consisted of testing and determining the effectiveness of the African American Health Belief Inventory on two samples—African Americans and European Americans—with similar duration of non-insulin-dependent, diabetes and similar age, sex, and socieconomic standing. Quantitative data from the AAHBI were integrated with qualitative interviews to produce a holistic view of the sociodemographic, psychosocial, and cultural factors that influence the African American diabetic health care-seeking pattern.

Stage 1: Qualitative Observations and Informal Interviews

The first stage of my diabetes study consisted only of observations and informal interviews of patients, physicians, and staff members in the Diabetes Clinic, beginning June 11, 1991. Once I arrived at the clinic (8:30a.m.), I immediately began my observations. From 8:30 a.m. to 12:00 p.m., I made the following physical observations of the site:

1. The Diabetes Clinic is located on the second floor of the Regenstrief Health Center;
2. The Diabetes Clinic is situated closely between two other clinics operating on the second floor;
3. The nurse/staff area is located in the center of the clinic (receptionist counter);
4. Patients must check in at the receptionist counter (nurse/staff central desk);
5. Patient waiting area is located on the right side of the clinic;
6. Patient waiting area seats a maximum of fifteen patients;
7. Patient waiting area has a limited number of magazines and no diabetes educational material on display;
8. Behind the receptionist desk are three major components of the clinic: the cubicles, the outpatient rooms, and the physicians' office;
9. Cubicles are the place for blood drawing and nurse/patient counseling;
10. Outpatient rooms are the place for diagnosis and treatment by the physician; and
11. Physicians' office is a place for the team of senior and junior physicians to examine patient charts.

In addition to the observations of the clinic, I conducted informal interviews with patients, physicians, nurses, and staff members during this first day. The following points best describe the major qualitative issues of concern to patients, physicians, and nurses:

1. Since physicians rotate to different clinics, patients rarely see the same physician twice;
2. Patients are often referred to another specialist and another clinic;
3. Patient adherence to prescribed diabetic regimen is very low;
4. Patients often arrive with family member or friend;
5. Patient's perception of their diabetes is often different from what the physician has told them;
6. Physicians expect degrees of difficulty for patients to adhere to diabetic regimen.

On this first day, for example, informal interviews with two patients highlighted their predicament and strategies for adhering to the diabetic regimen. While sitting in the patient area, I started a conversation with a middle-aged African American female (patient informant #1). After I informed her of my study, she agreed to share her story with me. Her story is summarized as follows:

Patient Informant #1: Patient informant #1 discovered her diabetic condition by accident. It happened when she cut her foot accidentally. After several weeks passed, her foot did not heal properly. She sought care from her regular doctor, and he diagnosed her diabetes. She was later referred to this Diabetes Clinic. Although she knew that other family members had developed diabetes, she did not think that she was susceptible. Patient informant #1 also felt that she did not need any assistance in her daily activities but later had to admit that she needed help from family members. Since her son lives with her, her daughter lives next door, and she has close friends in the neighborhood, she expressed a high degree of support from her network of family members and friends. Her motto is to, "live each day one day at a time."

Similarly, I conducted an informal interview with patient informant #2. After I explained the goal of my study, this middle-aged African American male agreed to share his story with me. His story is summarized as follows:

Patient Informant #2: Patient informant #2 was very apprehensive and suspicious of the doctors who treated him. He did not really trust them simply because his past relationship with doctors had been poor. He stated that the previous doctors did not tell him of the seriousness of his diabetes, so he did not strictly follow their prescribed regimen. Therefore, his blood glucose level increased, and he later became insulin-dependent diabetic. By being insulin-dependent diabetic, patient informant #2 must take insulin by injection. He hates the needle and the entire procedure for taking insulin through injection. He feels that it's demeaning to him. Yet, today, he is committed to following the doctor's orders and the diabetic regimen. He is a proud African American male who wants to maintain his dignity. Now that he asks more questions and takes an active part in adhering to the diabetic regimen, he feels that he can maintain his dignity and live longer.

By 12:27 p.m., I had completed my first day of observations and informal interviews at the Diabetes Clinic. This day was typical of all the remaining site visits that I conducted during the next five months.

From the nine total site visits over the five months, the following themes were significant with regard to the African American diabetic patient:

1. Assess the patient's cause of the diabetes;
2. Attempt to dispel any misconceptions of diabetes;
3. Activate the patient for self-care of diabetes;
4. Continue to reeducate the patient on blood glucose monitoring and insulin injection; and
5. Encourage social and familial support for adherence to diabetic regimen.

In addition, other qualitative results indicated that physicians need to (1) understand the sociocultural constraints of a patient's keeping appointments; (2) adjust the dietary modification of the patient to his or her lifestyle and ethnic dietary pattern; (3) develop more continuity of care; (4) learn new skills to develop rapport and trust with patients; and (5) emphasize the seriousness of the diabetic condition to the patient.

In conclusion, the qualitative results from stage 1 of this study helped to provide preliminary evidence that there was a definite need to further investigate the African American patient's diabetic regimen.

Stage 2: Qualitative Observations and Semi-Structured Interviews

Stage 2 consisted of conducting qualitative and quantitative observations and interviews of African American and Euro-American diabetic patients. For example, during the three-month portion of stage 2, African American patients shared the following comments:

Patient Informant #3: (African American male) *I believe that my diabetes is due to the stress that I endure each and every day. My lifestyle is uncertain and unpredictable, so I think that the stress that I am under caused my diabetes.*

Although patient informant #3 acknowledged that his eating pattern, lack of exercise, and overweight may have contributed to his current state of diabetes, he feels much more strongly that stress was the major reason.

Blacks have a predisposition to diabetes due to our heredity, but it is the stress in our lives that is of most importance.

Patient Informant #22: (African American male) *I really don't know what caused my diabetes. I have received a lot of explanations over the years, but I am still unsure of the actual cause.*

Patient Informant #8: (African American female) *I'm not sure what caused my diabetes. I know that there is a family connection to diabetes and my weight has something to do with it, but I don't take all of it too seriously.*

When asked to assess her ability to follow the doctor's prescribed diabetic dietary regimen, patient informant #8 stated:

My sons and husband want their meals the way they normally have it. They don't want no unseasoned meals, so what am I supposed to do?

Patient Informant #16: (African American female) *I was on those diabetic pills, but I had to be placed on insulin injections. I hate taking these injections, but I have to do it.*

Interestingly, patient informant #16 was placed on diabetic pills and told to watch her diet years ago. However, she stopped taking the pills on a regular basis and did not adhere to the diabetic diet regimen. Now that she is on insulin injections and closely adhering to the diabetes dietary regimen, her insulin injections have gradually been reduced.

Patient Informant #4: (African American male) *I was really not shocked when I was diagnosed with diabetes simply because my father and aunt have diabetes and I knew it was a matter of time before I would develop it.*

Diabetes is common among African Americans and this is due to our dietary eating pattern — fried foods and not enough vegetables.

Although patient informant #4 felt that it was a matter of time before he would develop diabetes, he is still unsure of the process and the reasons he developed type II diabetes. He came to the clinic only to find out what was wrong with his stomach. To his surprise, he was diagnosed with type II diabetes.

With regard to adherence to the diabetic regimen, patient informant #4 stated that African Americans would be able to follow closely the doctor's suggestions only if more basic information is told to them regarding the factors that influence one's diabetic condition. He stated the following as to the reason why he follows his diabetic regimen:

I would rather take the pills for my diabetes and live a long life than not take the pills and live a short, difficult life.

Interestingly, the qualitative results associated with the African American patients were quite similar to the qualitative findings associated with the Euro-American diabetic patients. The patient's lifestyle and occupation greatly influenced whether or not he or she could adhere to the prescribed diabetic regimen.

The qualitative findings that tended to be more associated with the African American diabetic patients than the Euro-American diabetic patients were as follows:

1. The uncertainty of the actual cause of one's diabetes;
2. The lack of perceived seriousness of one's diabetic condition;
3. The perceived inability to adhere to the diabetic regimen;
4. The lower ranking of one's health in comparison to other social and familial obligations.

These qualitative results indicated that a number of sociocultural issues still needed to be further investigated in the African American diabetic population.

Stage 3: Quantitative Interviews and Analyses of the AAHBI

Stage 3 consisted of testing and evaluating a culturally sensitive semistructured questionnaire (AAHBI) to be used in a clinical setting to assess the health beliefs and health care-seeking pattern of the African American diabetes patients. A comparison sample of Euro-Americans with similar duration of diabetes and similar, age, sex, and socioeconomic status was also interviewed.

The quantitative data were gathered from the questionnaire and entered into the mainframe computers at Indiana University/Purdue University Computer Center. The statistical package SPSS was used to analyze the data. The data analyses sought to determine the factors related to perceptions of diabetes, symptoms related to treatment for diabetes, health care-seeking behavior, and adherence to the diabetic regimen. Standard parametric statistics such as t-test, Pearson correlations, and multiple regressions were used to support the findings.

The sociodemographics of this study's sample were as follows:

A.   Ethnic Background
     1. African Americans (40%)
     2. Euro-Americans (56%)
     3. Other (4%)
B.   Gender
     1. Males (68%)
     2. Females (32%)
C.   Educational Background
     1. High School Education or equivalent (48%)
     2. Less than a high school education (30%)
     3. College Education (22%)
D.   Total sample = 25 patients

The quantitative analyses found a number of significant differences between African American and Euro-American diabetes patients in relation to their diabetic regimen. The significant differences were:

1.   African Americans (70%) were more more likely than Euro-Americans (35%) to agree that their diabetes is well controlled (p = .02).
2.   Euro-Americans (100%) were more likely than African Americans (60%) to disagree with the statement, "I cannot understand what the doctor told me about my diet/medication/ and diabetes" (p = .03).
3.   African Americans (50%) were less likely than Euro-Americans (14%) to recognize diabetes-related symptoms (p = .05).
4.   Euro-Americans (100%) were more likely than African Americans (80%) to believe that excess weight is related to diabetes (p = .05).
5.   African Americans (50%) were more likely than Euro-Americans (14%) to seek care at the clinic for their diabetes (p = .05).
6.   African Americans (50%) were more likely than Euro-Americans (7%) to join a support group for their diabetes (p = .03).
7.   Euro-Americans (81%) were more likely than African Americans (20%) to know their blood sugar count when arriving for a scheduled visit to the Diabetes Clinic (p = .03).

PHASE 4: REFLECTIVE COMMENTS

In this two-year applied medical anthropology study, the cultural health beliefs and health care-seeking pattern of African American diabetic patients influenced significantly individuals' degree of adherence to their diabetic regimen. The combination of the quantitative and the qualitative data indicates that African Americans experience uncertainty about their diabetic condition. In one respect, African Americans believed that they were well controlled and felt that they understood what the doctor told them about their diabetes. On the other hand, qualitative data (personal statements from patient informants) stated that there was a high degree of uncertainty about the cause of one's diabetes and how to treat it. In addition, African American diabetic patients tend not to be aware of the symptoms related to diabetes; tend not to know their blood sugar levels; and tend not to know the major factors associated with the development of diabetes.

The next question is Why don't African American patients know more about their diabetes? As indicated from the quantitative data, the answer is that African Americans honestly believe that they have received enough information from health care professionals and friends to take control of their diabetes. Thus, it is not that the African American patient was not being told about his or her diabetic condition; rather, the lack of adherence to the diabetic regimen relates more to the lack of understanding between the two parties (patient and health care professional) when they discuss the patient's diabetic condition. Both parties felt that they understood each other, but in actuality, they did not. This lack of understanding results in the poor adherence to the diabetic regimen among African Americans. With the implementation of the African American Health Belief Inventory, we were able to highlight the major sociocultural factors as to why so many African American diabetes patients experienced difficulty in adhering to the diabetic regimen.

Interestingly, the findings from this study were quite similar to those of Uzoma and Feldman's (1989) study of African American diabetic patients attending an inner-city teaching hospital outpatient clinic in Washington, DC. Uzoma and Feldman found that cost and lack of information were indicated by African American female patients as a barrier to insulin adherence. In addition, they recommended that (1) self-efficacy training be utilized for the entire patient population, (2) programs be tailored to specific gender and age groups, and (3) use of social support should be encouraged for female patients. Finally, since diabetes control and insulin adherence have not been addressed adequately within the African American community, Uzoma and Feldman suggested that intense, well-targeted, community-based, and culturally appropriate outreach and education programs be developed to reach African American patients.

CONCLUSION

The primary aim of this applied medical anthropology project was to assess the cultural health beliefs and health care-seeking pattern of African American and Euro-American diabetes patients. A secondary objective was to construct a clinical/cultural assessment tool–the African American Health Belief Inventory.

The quantitative and qualitative findings indicated that it is vitally important to assess the following health care issues concerning the African American diabetes patients:

1.   perceived cause of their diabetes;
2.   the lifestyle and dietary pattern of each patient; and
3.   the perceived seriousness of the diabetic condition to the patient.

All three of these health care issues influence greatly the ability of the African American patient to adhere to the prescribed diabetic regimen.

POST-EVALUATION QUESTIONS

1.   Describe how you would have improved this applied medical anthropology fieldwork project.

2.   Discuss the type of cultural health interventions that you would implement for this particular population.

3.   Are there any other health, social or cultural issues that need to be addressed to assist other health care professionals when working with the African American diabetes population?

REFERENCES

Bailey, Eric. 1991. *Urban African American Health Care*. Lanham, MD: University Press of America.

Drury, T.F. et al. 1985. "Sociodemographics Characteristics of Adult Diabetes." In *Diabetes in America*. Washington DC: US Government Printing Office. NIH Publication No. 85-1468.

Glascow, Russell and Deborah Toobert. 1988. "Social Environment and Regimen Adherence among Type II Diabetic Patients." *Diabetes Care* 11: 377–386.

Gohdes, Dorothy. 1988. "Diet Therapy for Minority Patients with Diabetes." *Diabetes Care* 11: 189–191.

Harris, M. et al. 1987. "Prevalence of Diabetes and Impaired Glucose Tolerance and Plasma Glucose Levels in U.S. Population Aged 20-74 Years." *Diabetes* 36: 523–534.

Interagency State Council on Black and Minority Health. 1992. *Assessing Indi-ana's Black and Minority Health Status.* Indianapolis: Indiana State Health Department.

Otten, M. W.,. Jr., Teutsch SM, Williamson DF, Mark, JS. 1990. "The Effect of Known Risk Factors on the Excess Mortality of Black Adults in the United States." *Journal of the American Medical Association* 263: 845–850.

Ruderman, Neil et al. 1990. "Exercise in Therapy and Prevention of Type II Diabetes." *Diabetes Care* 13: 1163–1168.

Tjoa, Hong and Norman Kaplan. 1991. "Nonpharmacological Treatment of Hy-pertension in Diabetes Mellitus." *Diabetes Care* 14: 449–460.

U.S. Department of Health and Human Services. 1986. "Diabetes in Black Americans." In *Report of the Secretary's Task Force on Black and Mi-nority Health.* Pp. 214–218. Washington, DC:US Government Printing Office.

———. 1990. *Institute of Diabetes and Digestive and Kidney Disease (NIDDK)* NIH Publication No. 90-1585. Washington, DC:US Government Printing Office.

Uzoma, Catherine and Robert Feldman. 1989. "Psychosocial Factors Influenc-ing Inner City Black Diabetic Patients Adherence with Insulin." *Health Education* 20: 29–32.

Wagenknect, Lynne et al. 1989. "Epidemiology of IDDM in Black and White Children in Jefferson County, Alabama, 1979–1985." *Diabetes* 38: 629–633.

WEB SITES OF SIGNIFICANCE

American Diabetes Association

http://www.diabetes.org

National Center for Chronic Disease Prevention and Health Promotion

http://www.cdc.gov/nccdphp/nccdhome.htm

National Institute of Diabetes and Digestive and Kidney Diseases

http://www.niddk.nih.gov/

Chapter 13

HIV/AIDS Counseling and the African American Community

CRITICAL THINKING QUESTIONS

1. Why is it important to conduct fieldwork on HIV/AIDS in the African American community?

2. Why is it important to understand the particular strategies of the HIV/AIDS counselor?

3. How does the African American community perceive HIV/AIDS?

INTRODUCTION

The objectives of this applied medical anthropology study were twofold: to examine the basic job functions and alternative strategies that HIV/AIDS case managers/counselors use to work with their clients and to develop new case manager/counselor guidelines for a culturally diverse HIV/AIDS population, particularly African Americans and Hispanic/Latino Americans. Focus groups of case managers/counselors were conducted at local HIV/AIDS organizations in the Atlanta area. From the case manager's focus group sessions, four major themes emerged: (1) case manager's roles and strategies; (2) HIV/AIDS health beliefs and attitudes; (3) family members/friends network issues and adaptive strategies; and (4) case manager's cultural intervention strategies. Given our understanding of the health beliefs and attitudes of HIV/AIDS in ethnic minority and sociocultural groups, the case manager/counselor's perspective provides unique insight and innovative strategies for public health interventions.

In order to critically examine the health beliefs and attitudes of HIV/AIDS in ethnic minority and sociocultural groups from the case manager/counselor perspective, this exploratory study undertook a unique approach of investigating

HIV/AIDS in the Atlanta metropolitan area. This approach involves examining HIV/AIDS from the HIV/AIDS case manager's (sometimes referred to as HIV/AIDS counselor's) perspective. The primary purpose of this research strategy was not only to recognize the role and skills of these special health care providers but also to understand the different strategies that these professionals use when working with their HIV/AIDS clients.

The three major objectives of this exploratory study, therefore, were: (1) to examine the basic job functions and alternative cultural strategies that HIV/AIDS case manager/counselors use to work with their clients; (2) to discover successful cultural intervention strategies that HIV/AIDS case managers/counselors use for their clientele; and (3) to develop new public health HIV/AIDS case manager/counselor guidelines for African American and Hispanic/Latino American populations.

BACKGROUND INFORMATION

HIV/AIDS: 1981–1990

The first cases of acquired immunodeficiency syndrome (AIDS) were recognized and described in 1981. During the 1980s, the number of reported AIDS cases increased each year. Homesexual/bisexual men and intravenous (IV) drug users have accounted for the largest number of AIDS cases throughout the epidemic. The total number of AIDS cases and of cases in these categories increased most rapidly during the middle 1980s, with more moderate increases in the late 1980s (Centers for Disease Control and Prevention 1986).

Reported AIDS cases associated with heterosexual transmission of human immunodeficiency virus (HIV) have been increasing steadily, with cases occurring more frequently among women than among men. Similarly, cases of children associated with perinatal (mother-to-infant) HIV transmission have continued to increase. The number of AIDS cases associated with blood or blood product transfusions has stabilized (Centers for Disease Control and Prevention 1986).

In 1990, 43,339 AIDS cases (17.2 per 100,00 population) were reported, accounting for more than one-fourth (161,073) of all cases reported during 1981—1990. Homosexual/bisexual men and IV drug users represented more than three-fourths of reported cases (Centers for Disease Control and Prevention 1993).

The number of cases reported per 100,000 population was higher for men, blacks, and Hispanics, persons 30–39 and 40–49 years of age, and persons in the U.S. territories and the Northeast than for persons in other demographic groups or geographic areas. Reported cases among both women and men varied widely among states (Centers for Disease Control and Prevention 1993).

HIV/AIDS: Racial & Ethnic Minority 1990s Data

Racial and ethnic minority populations have been disproportionately affected by HIV infection and AIDS since the beginning of the epidemic in the United States. In 1993, the Centers for Disease Control and Prevention received reports of 315,390 cases of AIDS among persons in the United States, including 97,794 cases among blacks, 52,531 among Hispanics, 2,036 among Asians/Pacific Islanders, and 657 among American Indians/Alaskan Natives. Through mid-1993, 48% of all reported AIDS cases were among blacks and Hispanics, while these two population groups represent only 21% of the total U.S. population. In 1991, HIV infection and AIDS were the sixth leading cause of death among blacks and seventh leading cause of death among Hispanics, while they ranked tenth among whites (Centers for Disease Control and Prevention 1993).

Minority women and children have been particularly hard hit. Of reported AIDS cases among adult and adolescent women, 74% are among blacks and Hispanics; among children (less than 13 years of age), 79% of cases are among blacks and Hispanics. Both the proportions of deaths and the death rates associated with HIV/AIDS are substantially higher for black and Hispanic women than for women in other racial/ethnic populations (Centers for Disease Control and Prevention 1993).

In addition, the rate of infection among black and Hispanic homosexual and bisexual males is two or three times higher than for their non-Hispanic white counterparts. Similarly, the same disproportionate rate of infection is evident when one compares white heterosexual and nonwhite heterosexual populations. Specifically, heterosexual transmission among Hispanics and blacks is linked to infection of drug users and their sexual partners. Among Hispanics, the infected population includes homosexual and bisexual men who are not injection drug users (53%) and heterosexual male injection drug users (35%) (Centers for Disease Control and Prevention 1993).

HIV/AIDS Counselors

In the evolution of HIV care, many types of professionals and laypersons have involved themselves in the task of counseling or case managing people living with HIV and AIDS. The terms "counseling" and "case-managing" must be broadly defined primarily because they can range from advice about access to health care and legal services to traditional forms of psychiatric treatment, including medical treatment of clinical depression. In addition, today counselors who work with HIV and AIDS clients have had varying degrees of training as mental health providers, and they include social workers, psychologists, psychiatrists, nurses, clergy, and lay peer counselors (Dworkin and Pincu 1993).

The qualifications for a counselor may vary, but at a minimum counselors should have

- a working knowledge of their clients' HIV disease process based on medical and nursing assessments;
- knowledge of, and contact with, services in immediate and neighboring communities, health care and social services agencies, and public entitlement programs;
- resourcefulness and creativity in accessing required services; and
- interpersonal skills that allow effective interaction with clients and multiple providers in the households, communities, and medical settings while maintaining a spirit of hope and empathy.

Finally, to be an effective counselor for persons with HIV disease, it is important to consider how social, cultural, and ethnic influences shape individuals' responses to illness and their health seeking behaviors in general (Medrano and Klopner 1992; Dworkin and Pincu 1993; Croteau, Nero, and Johnson 1993; Harwood 1981; Purcell et al. 1998). The Western medical model often overlooks "illness," or the individual's perception of what is wrong, in favor of sophisticated technical procedures and laboratory tests. This lack of attention to the individual's experience of the problem is particularly noticeable to the individual who is socially, culturally, and ethnically different. Once the individual counselor acknowledges and addresses these essential issues, the HIV/AIDS counselor can become more successful in working closely with clients.

PHASE 1: PREPARING AND ADAPTING TO THE FIELD

Since I had no previous background in the area of HIV/AIDS, I prepared myself for this applied medical anthropology project in three different ways. First, I enrolled in a college course at Emory University School of Public Health entitled, An Overview of HIV/AIDS. This course informed students of the medical and behavioral aspects of HIV/AIDS. Second, I conducted a thorough library research on as many aspects of HIV/AIDS that I could think of. Third, I conducted interviews with key public health administrators, physicians, and a person who was HIV positive to obtain a preliminary overview on how the city and state health care systems of Atlanta and Georgia truly addressed HIV/AIDS.

PHASE 2: MEDICAL ANTHROPOLOGY FIELDWORK TECHNIQUES

Overall, this project consisted of three stages: (1) qualitative interviews with key informants in the local health care system; (2) participant observations of HIV/AIDS support groups; and (3) qualitative interviews with HIV/AIDS counselors.

In August 1993, I began my qualitative interviews with key health care professional informants in the metropolitan Atlanta area. Additionally, I spoke with a person who was diagnosed HIV positive and who was very active in advocating support for those individuals and families affected by HIV/AIDS.

From June 1994 to August 1994, I observed and participated in two local, community-based HIV/AIDS support groups. Each group catered to a particular type of HIV/AIDS population. For instance, the HIV/AIDS organization located in downtown Atlanta catered more to a transient, homosexual/bisexual population, whereas the organization located fifteen miles northeast of Atlanta catered more to a heterosexual males who had been long-term residents of Atlanta.

Finally, stage 3 consisted of interviews of HIV/AIDS counselors at four different community-based HIV/AIDS organizations in the Atlanta metropolitan area. In particular, qualitative interviews (focus groups) concentrated upon the counselors who primarily worked with the African American and Hispanic/Latino HIV/AIDS population. The qualitative data gathered from the focus groups established the basis of the findings from this applied medical anthropology project.

PHASE 3: ETHNOGRAPHIC FIELDWORK DATA ANALYSES

Qualitative Analyses: The Health Care System and HIV/AIDS

The qualitative analyses from my interviews with five key health care professional individuals and their health care organization revealed valuable insight into the sociocultural-political factors that affect HIV/AIDS intervention in the Atlanta metropolitan area. The key informants were representatives of the following organizations: (1) Fulton County Health Department, (2) Fulton County's Tuberculosis clinic, (3) Dekalb-Grady clinic, (4) Morehouse School of Medicine AIDS Education Project, and (5) Georgia Women Preventing AIDS organization.

The qualitative information gathered from each key informant was intended to discover more than the "ideal" cultural patterning of each organization's services, the "real" cultural patterning and the significant issues that key informants felt about their organization.

Informant #1: Representative of Fulton County Health Department

This African American informant had served at Fulton County Health Department since 1978 and had witnessed a number of changes over the years. With regard to public health needs, Fulton County Health Department (F.C.H.D.) is responsible for the indigent in the county and collaborates with Grady Hospital for patient care. The Department of Health has twenty physical health clinics, four mental health clinics, and three mental retardation centers.

The informant indicated that Fulton County Health Department is actually under the authority of the county commissioners and not the State Health Department, thereby receiving most of its funding from Fulton County and not the state of Georgia. This type of funding arrangement was instituted by Georgia in 1954 or 1955.

This funding arrangement has influenced Fulton County to address more clinical care than preventive care for patients. Yet, due to the inability of Fulton County Health Department to make significant changes in health outcomes for Fulton County residents, my informant stated that more focus will be toward outreach programs such as HIV/AIDS and tuberculosis. The informant emphasized that Fulton County Health Department must attempt to develop more of a community involvement (empowerment) and mechanisms for coalition building. If these two future objectives are strongly implemented, then more preventive HIV/AIDS and tuberculosis education can reach those who care and follow up.

Informant #2: Representative of Fulton County's Tuberculosis Clinic

This African American informant had served as medical director of the Tuberculosis Clinic for only one year. Yet her association with Fulton County Health Department had been for approximately eleven years. During the past eleven years, her job responsibilities have changed frequently because of the changing administration and priorities of the Department.

In her current position with F.C.H.D., this informant felt that its administration experienced too much bureaucracy and that often current policy may affect the manner in which the department can provide effective tuberculosis and HIV services for its clientele. She emphasized that her position was primarily created because of the politics at F.C.H.D. and the pressure from local health administrators to do something about the local tuberculosis epidemic. F.C.H.D. therefore assigned her to the tuberculosis medical officer position.

This informant felt strongly that one of the major problems with patient care is the patient. She stated that it is the "patient's responsibility to find out which specialist to care for them and which agency to seek services from as it relates to their tuberculosis or HIV/AIDS."

She concluded our interview by stating that, "the patient should educate themselves and take advantage of the advanced technology for their health."

Informant #3: Dekalb Grady Clinic

This African American informant physician works at this South Dekalb neighborhood health clinic. Since she had received her training via a federally supported grant, she felt committed to work at a community-based health clinic. She had worked at the Dekalb Grady Cinic for ten to twelve years.

Being a very socially conscious minded physician, this informant stated that a large percentage of her patients tended to fall through the cracks and get lost in the system. She emphasized that it is very difficult to follow patients from her clinic to a local hospital simply because there is virtually no collaboration or connection of record keeping or chart analyses of a patient's history. In fact, she stated that some of her patients had never been notified by this local hospital that they had tested positive for HIV several years ago.

This informant emphasized that "we must try to keep patients into the health system and attempt to coordinate better use of our services from clinic to hospital."

Informant # 4: Morehouse School of Project Medicine AIDS Education

This African American informant was the director of the Morehouse School of Medicine AIDS Education Project. She stated that the African American community has not seriously addressed the HIV/AIDS epidemic. In fact, she emphasized that a large percentage of the African American ministers have not yet discussed HIV in their congregations and neighborhoods. However, in conjunction with the support from other local organizations in the community, local African American churches were beginning to develop new HIV/AIDS outreach initiatives.

Informant #5: The Georgia Women Preventing AIDS

As a spokesperson for the Georgia Women Preventing AIDS organization and as an HIV positive person, this African American woman provided in-depth and practical aspects to individuals who are affected by AIDS. She felt that the HIV/AIDS message must continue to be promoted and marketed for the public—particularly for women of all cultural and ethnic backgrounds who are disfranchised and who lack empowerment.

This informant felt strongly that having safer sexual practices is a priority and a "must" for all women. She realized that her approach of constantly talking openly about HIV and sexual practices may offend some people, yet if the message reached one individual in the audience, she felt that she had accomplished her job.

When asked, "How do you continue to do outreach education, and how do you continue to get the strength to do your job?" She simply stated, "The Lord!"

Overall, the preliminary qualitative data gathered from the five informants helped me to obtain a better understanding of the "real cultural patterning" among those who work in local health care system and those who were personally affected by HIV/AIDS.

Qualitative Analyses of Community-Based HIV/AIDS Support Groups

To better understand the social and cultural issues that the HIV counselor encountered, I participated in two HIV/AIDS community-based support groups. My key informants from each organization had invited me to observe and to participate in the support group sessions. Before each session began, my key informants introduced me and informed the group that I was present to learn from them.

The first HIV/AIDS support group in which I participated was called Common Ground. Common Ground is located in downtown Atlanta near Piedmont Park and the Playhouse theater. Upstairs in a two-story house were the offices for Common Ground and Interfaith Agencies, which kept Common Ground operating. On the first floor were the meeting room, staff offices, waiting area, and kitchen. Common Ground functioned as a meeting place and social support network for HIV positive individuals. Its clientele consisted primarily of gay white males and females, and gay African American males and females.

On February 2, 1995, I participated in my first support group session at Common Ground. The support group session started about 11:00 a.m.. The total number of individuals was approximately fifteen. At the beginning of this session, my key informant stated that the goal for the day's session was to provide social support meditation and discussion.

Once all the participants had arrived, we moved to the living room area and took our seats in a circular formation. After introductions, the HIV counselor asked us to pray. We were then asked to look through the piles of newspapers on the center table and to design a picture that depicts the individual's representation of a "safe place." After all of us completed this assignment, each of us stood up and explained why we had selected our design.

The primary purpose of this group exercise was to allow each individual to show his or her personality and to visualize what a "safe place" meant to that individual. As the HIV counselor emphasized, it is important for an HIV positive individual to visualize what a "safe place" really looks like. Interestingly, the entire support group's pictures showed similar themes.

After our group picture exercise, each person shared his or her personal experience with HIV. I shared a story of a family member who was diagnosed with HIV. Each story revealed the levels of adjustment and adaptation that all of us had endured when discussing the topic of HIV/AIDS.

A number of common issues were shared: (1) individual denial of gay status, (2) family members' denial of the individual's gay status, (3) fear of rejection from family members and friends, (4) final acceptance of gay status and HIV positive status, and (5) development of a new support system. The major themes from these stories were (1) having faith in the Lord, (2) thinking positive, (3) gaining stages of awareness and acceptance of HIV, and (4) finding a safe place.

The second HIV/AIDS support group in which I participated was the AID Gwinnett County support group. AID Gwinnett Inc. is a not-for-profit, community-based organization incorporated in Gwinnett County in October 1991. The organization responds on a grassroots level to HIV/AIDS epidemic within their community—Gwinnett, Rockdale, Newton, and surrounding northeast Atlanta areas. AID Gwinnett provides services, resources, education, advocacy, and support to people living with HIV/AIDS. Through collaborative efforts between the community, other services, and support agencies—both governmental and private—AID Gwinnett provides direct services to PWAs (Persons with AIDS) and acts as an educational resource to promote awareness of the nature and impact of HIV/AIDS.

On February 14, 1995, I participated in AID Gwinnett's support group session. The support group session began at 7:30 p.m. and lasted approximately an hour and a half. There were twelve individuals in this session, including myself. A majority were men from various social, cultural, and lifestyle backgrounds. Additionally, most men were heterosexual and married.

The group moderator introduced me as an observer to this support group session and asked each individual to share his or her story as in every other session prior to my arrival. Within seconds, individuals began to share their stories and share their feelings on how they had arrived at their current state of adjusting to being HIV+.

From each personal story, there were four common themes:

1. the HIV+ person usually tells a friend before the family;
2. the HIV+ person must prepare himself or herself mentally to tell the family;
3. the HIV+ person must give the family time and patience in coping with the concept of HIV and AIDS; and
4. the HIV+ person and family undergo phases of understanding and adapting to HIV/AIDS.

Qualitative Analyses of HIV/AIDS Counselor Focus Groups

There were two focus groups conducted in ethnic minority communities— St. Joseph Hispanic Health Services and SisterLove, Inc.. St. Joseph's Hispanic Health Services, located at Mercy Mobile Health Care facility, was founded in 1987 to serve the Atlanta metropolitan community. Special services and program activities were also developed for the Hispanic/Latino community. Culturally and linguistically appropriate Hispanic/Latino programs included prenatal programs, social services programs, educational programs, substance abuse prevention program for Hispanic/Latino adolescents, and HIV/STD (sexually transmitted disease) programs.

SisterLove, Inc. is a nonprofit organization established to increase the knowledge and practice of preventive health in relation to HIV infection and AIDS in communities where women are at risk or already living with HIV/AIDS. It is the goal of SisterLove to instill education and empowerment in women at risk and HIV+ women in and around metropolitan Atlanta. The project's programs include an educator's bureau, facilitator training, target outreach, program development assistance, self-help group development, a support group program, Love House Supportive Living Residence, and the "Healthy Love Party," a safer sex workshop for women. While SisterLove, Inc., recognizes and addresses the needs of all women, African American women, the most affected population among women with AIDS, receive particular attention within all their culturally appropriate programs.

St. Joseph Hispanic Health Services Themes and Patterns

In this counselor focus group session, five major themes emerged:

1. counselor's roles and strategies;
2. HIV+ health beliefs and attitudes;
3. perceptions of local mainstream health care system;
4. Hispanic/Latino family cultural patterns; and
5. Hispanic/Latino HIV+ counselor cultural intervention strategies.

Initial discussion of the focus group centered around the issues of Hispanics/Latinos' perception of the local mainstream health care system. Counselors emphasized that the clients they see, as well as the Hispanic/Latino community at large, tend not to trust the system for health care or social services. Although many of their HIV+ clients and non-HIV+ clients use the local health care system periodically, they tend not to stay with particular health care or social programs due to three major factors: (1) the clients' or family members' document status (U.S. citizenship) may be in question; (2) there is a lack of bicultural/bilingual HIV counselors and health care professionals; and (3) local health care and social systems are not culturally designed for Hispanics/Latinos. These issues were discussed and emphasized by the focus group participants before specific issues regarding counselor strategies for HIV clients.

Among the Hispanic/Latina focus group counselors, each was specialized for a particular segment of the Hispanic/Latino community—one counselor worked specifically with adolescents; one counselor worked specifically with HIV drug users; and one counselor worked as an HIV/AIDS family coordinator. Regardless of their HIV specialty area, all counselors agreed upon basic job functions:

1. to evaluate basic and essential needs of the HIV+ client;
2. to acknowledge the "feelings" of the HIV+ client;
3. to connect HIV+ clients with their community organization or local church; and
4. to implement basic educational enrichment programs.

The focus group also discussed the "cultural function" of their job responsibilities and cultural awareness skills as Hispanic/Latina counselors. These particular cultural patterns were described as follows:

- Respect is a priority with Hispanics.
- Hispanic parents will respect authority figures (teachers, health care professionals.
- The family must be taken into account for every health intervention, including the large extended family.
- Health beliefs must be respected.

- HIV/AIDS and Gay/Lesbian issues directly conflict with the Hispanic family orientation.
- If male (husband) is HIV positive, the woman (wife) would also want to be positive otherwise guilt and shame on the family.
- If the woman is HIV positive, the male (husband) has to be HIV positive, otherwise extreme guilt and shame on the family.
- The more assimilated the Latina women, the more likely substance abuse may occur.

The Hispanic/Latina counselors stated that the preceding cultural patterns and beliefs show the importance of this issue to the average Hispanic/Latino client. Highlighting these few cultural issues enables other counselors to be more aware of the true impact and significance of cultural health beliefs and care issues to job performance and effectiveness in the Hispanic/Latino community.

Furthermore, these cultural job function issues related directly to Hispanic/Latino Americans' HIV/AIDS health beliefs and attitudes. Focus group members indicated that HIV/AIDS health beliefs and attitudes such as *stigma, denial, shame, and delay* all influence the HIV+ clients and their family/friends network in not seeking early prevention and counseling advice from HIV counselors.

In fact, according to one of the counselors, "it is customary to expect that those who eventually arrive at the HIV clinic for counseling usually are in the latter stages of HIV/AIDS." Despite this pattern of seeking care in the latter stages of the disease, the focus group stressed that it will continue to find new ways to reach its clients and families as early as possible with HIV prevention material.

Finally, the focus group highlighted a number of HIV cultural intervention strategies that should be considered for the Hispanic/Latino client and community:

1. Conduct frequent home visits;
2. Involve the whole family in any HIV education intervention;
3. Acknowledge the importance of health beliefs to the client and the family;
4. Find out the individual's and the family's country of origin, reasons for arrival in the United States language pattern, educational level, and number of years in the United States; and
5. Be prepared to develop interventions for the HIV+ clients in their latter stages of the disease.

The focus group reiterated that the aforementioned Hispanic/Latino cultural interventions were directly related to the basic elements of Hispanic/Latino culture. The focus group described these basic cultural patterns as follows:

1. Men and women's roles are clearly defined;
2. Men tend to be the major decision makers;
3. Hispanics/Latinos prefer to have large families;

4. Children were strongly desired; and
5. Hispanic/Latino culture tends to be more "relaxed" and less rigid/structured than the American culture.

SisterLove, Inc./AID Atlanta Themes and Patterns

From the counselors' focus group session, five themes emerged: (1) counselor roles and strategies; (2) African American women's HIV+ health beliefs and attitudes; (3) African American women's support group issues; (4) African American family/friends network and adaptation; and (5) counselor cultural intervention strategies.

The counselor's major job responsibilities with an HIV+ client is (1) to develop a "care plan"—essential needs such as food, clothing, housing, income, and social support are evaluated; (2) to connect an HIV+ client with other social and health agencies in the community; and (3) to prioritize the basic needs of the client.

In order to be even more successful with their HIV+ African American clients, the counselors stated that it is very important to develop a good partnership with the client and to empower the client to be the decision maker of the HIV+ lifestyle. By following the counselor strategy for their clients, the focus group felt that the African American women whom they served could better adapt to some of the actual and perceived barriers from society at large and from their family, social, and friend network.

In fact, the focus group stated that the support group is the place where African American women (HIV/AIDS clients and counselors) hear of other African American women's attitudes and beliefs about HIV. The African American women's support group is therefore a place to hear about individual and group adaptation to their HIV/AIDS status.

For example, the focus group stated that "a lot of women do not tell their partners." The major reasons many African American women do not tell their partners or family members about being HIV+ include, but are not limited to, the following:

1. Don't know if partner is going to be HIV+.
2. Punish me.
3. Try to protect others from the situation.
4. Women are taught to take care of everyone else. I'm always okay. I'm always going to be here.
5. So many other things to take care of—children, food, housing, and income.
6. Don't want to burden others.
7. Women internalize and keep it in.

The African American women's HIV+ support group also helps women to address a number of HIV related issues such as misconceptions of HIV, acknowledgment of HIV+ status to family/friends; and family involvement. In fact, one counselor stated, "Once family members come, they do see a different aspect of their HIV+ family member."

According to the focus group, however, family members are usually told last about the HIV status of their family member and are often reluctant to accept and work with their family member. Responses of the counselors about the HIV+ client's family range from denial of the HIV+ status, to denial of the individual's possible drug addiction or gay/lesbian lifestyle, to perception that the government cannot be trusted regarding information on the transmission of the virus.

By recognizing and accepting the patterns of adaptation of HIV+ clients and their families, the counselors suggested following cultural intervention strategies for the African American women:

1. Realize that most of the women will not tell others of their HIV status due to the perceived consequences from their partners/spouse/family members;
2. Pose a question or a scenario in order for clients to assess critically their situation and begin discussing their HIV/AIDS status openly;
3. Encourage HIV/AIDS clients to participate in small support group discussions;
4. Accept where people are and praise their achievements; and
5. Connect clients with other African American cultural institutions such as the local church, community center, and social organization in their community.

PHASE FOUR: REFLECTIVE COMMENTS

The major results of the two focus group sessions, the observation of HIV support groups, and qualitative interviews of community health professionals helped to provide insight about the major health care issues related to HIV/AIDS counseling. They were (1) counselor basic job functions; (2) counselor cultural job intervention strategies; (3) recognition of client's HIV/AIDS health beliefs and attitudes; and (4) HIV/AIDS public health strategies.

The qualitative observations and interviews of the HIV/AIDS counselor emphasized the definite need to further investigate this relatively new area of HIV/AIDS intervention—HIV/AIDS counseling. In fact, very few research studies have been conducted in this area from a public health, medical anthropological approach. The qualitative observations and results of this exploratory study, therefore, become more significant for public health professionals as they recognize the need to develop new HIV counseling procedures and prevention programs for the public.

In order to assist counselors with their ethnic and socioculturally diverse HIV/AIDS population, this exploratory study recommends seven key points:

1. Counselors must become familiar with group-specific, HIV/AIDS-related misconceptions and attitudes;

2. Counselors need new HIV/AIDS guidelines for cross-cultural and intra group intervention;
3. Counselors need to develop new strategies to include the family/friends network of the HIV/AIDS client;
4. Family members/friends need to work closely with HIV/AIDS counselors to better understand the lifestyle adaptation of the HIV/AIDS individual;
5. Counselors need new national counselor guidelines for the ethnic minority and culturally diverse HIV/AIDS population;
6. Counselors need new national training procedures for HIV/AIDS counselors; and
7. Researchers need to develop new national qualitative and quantitative tools for the counselors to better understand the lifestyle and adaptive processes of their HIV/AIDS clients.

CONCLUSION

The framework of this project originates from two major fields of study—medical anthropology and public health. The collaboration of these two disciplines for the purpose of investigating this critical health care issue of HIV/AIDS in ethnic minority populations shows how behavioral and social science can play a significant role in HIV/AIDS health care research.

The importance of behavioral and social science research to the study of the HIV/AIDS epidemic is embodied in the following statement from the Committee for a National Strategy for AIDS:

Social science research can play a number of valuable roles in meeting the challenge of AIDS. It can help in the development of effective education programs to encourage changes in behavior that will break the chain of HIV transmission. It can contribute to the development of informed public policies that reduce the public's fear of AIDS and discriminatory practices towards AIDS sufferers. And it can guide the establishment of improved health care and social services that further the ability to treat AIDS patients effectively, humanely, and at reasonable cost. Such research can be useful in guiding short-term administrative and social responses to the epidemic and in providing the clarification necessary for developing longer-term measures for coping with AIDS and, more generally, with future health crises (Institute of Medicine National Academy of Sciences 1986: 265).

POST-EVALUATION QUESTIONS

1. How would you have improved this applied medical anthropological project?

2. How can understanding the cultural beliefs of HIV/AIDS among African Americans help health care professionals work better with their clients?

3. How does the local health care system affect the implementation of HIV/AIDS programs for the African American community?

REFERENCES

Centers for Disease Control and Prevention. 1993. *Facts about HIV/AIDS and Race/ethnicity*. Atlanta: U.S. Government Printing Office.

Croteau J., C. Nero, and D. Johnson. 1993. "Social and Cultural Sensivity in Group Specific HIV and AIDS programming." *Journal of Counseling & Development*, 71: 290–296.

Dignan, M. and P. Carr. 1992. *Program Planning for Health Education and Promotion*. Second. ed. Philadelphia: Lea and Febiger.

Dworkin S., and L. Pincu. 1993. "Counseling in the era of AIDS." *Journal of Counseling and Development* 71: 275–281.

Harwood, A. 1981. "Guidelines for Culturally Appropriate Health Care." In *Ethnicity and Medical Care*. A. Harwood, ed. Pp. 483–507. Cambridge, MA: Harvard University Press.

Institute of Medicine National Academy of Sciences. 1986. *Confronting AIDS: Directions for Public Health, Health Care and Research*. Washington, DC: National Academy Press.

Leininger, M. 1985. *Qualitative Research Methods in Nursing*. New York: Grune and Stratton, Inc.

Medrano L. and M. Klopner. 1992. "AIDS and People of Color." In *AIDS: A Complete Guide to Psychosocial Intervention*. L. Medrano and M. Klopner, eds. Pp. 117–139. Milwaukee: Family Service America.

Purcell, David et al. 1998. "HIV Prevention Case Management: Current Practice and Future Directions." *Health and Social Work* 23: 282–289.

WEB SITES OF SIGNIFICANCE

National Center for HIV, STD, and Tuberculosis Prevention

http://www.cdc.gov/nchstp/od/nchstp.html

Office AIDS Research

http://www.cdc.gov/nchstp/od/nchstp.html

Chapter 14

A Community's Perception
of the Health Care System:
Issues of Equity

CRITICAL THINKING QUESTIONS

1. Why is it important to conduct fieldwork on issues of health care equity within the African American community?

2. What can the medical anthropologist learn from studying issues of equity?

3. How does the African American community perceive equity of health care in the community?

INTRODUCTION

The primary aim of this study was to assess the cultural attitude of the local health care system among African Americans in two counties of Indiana. With the cooperation and assistance of the Indiana State Health Department and local African Americans, a qualitative and quantitative study was conducted. Eleven focus groups, five individual, in-depth interviews, and 101 surveys were used to collect the cultural attitudinal data as they relate to health care utilization patterns. Qualitative and quantitative data analyses indicate that there were four significant attitudinal differences between the African American focus groups and the control group. In addition, socioeconomic and intragenerational factors influenced the cultural attitude of African Americans toward the local health care system.

When health care researchers analyze a population's health care utilization pattern, it is important to distinguish between the concepts of health needs and wants and the demand for health services. A population's need for services may be determined by either normative medical judgments or individually perceived needs.

Wants refer to the number of health services that individuals feel they ought to consume, based on their own perceptions of their health needs. *Demand* is the number of health services that individuals wish to consume at specified prices, using available financial resources and considering preferences for all other goods and services.

Utilization is the actual number of services consumed when demand is translated into care-seeking behavior. Individuals' wants may be more or less than their needs or demands for care.

These distinctions are important because they underlie notions of equity in, and relative shortages of, health services. Equity assumes that services are provided to meet everyone's need for care, as determined by either professional medical judgments or the self-perceptions of the public. Failure to achieve equity may be the result of shortages in personnel, facilities, and other resources, or it may be due to a lack of understanding of wants and needs of the population being served (Bailey 1991, 1994).

In order to examine the issues of equity of health care in Indiana, this study investigated primarily one major health care issue—"What social and cultural factors (attitudes, beliefs, and values) affect African Americans' use of health care services in two counties in Indiana? The three major objectives of this study were as follows:

1.   to examine the cultural attitudes, beliefs, and values of African American residents in St. Joseph and Allen counties;
2.   to determine the relationship of cultural attitudes, beliefs, and values to health care-seeking options and prenatal care at local health facilities; and
3.   to determine the relationship of cultural attitudes, beliefs, and values to health care behavior.

To reiterate, culture is a system of shared health beliefs, values, customs, and behaviors that are transmitted from generation to generation through learning. This learned health culture patterning guides health care action and health beliefs to meet both familiar and new illness situations.

BACKGROUND INFORMATION

Allen County

Allen County is located in the northeastern corner of Indiana, bordering Ohio. The third largest county in the state, Allen County has a population of 300,000. This represents 5.4% of the population. The racial composition of Allen county is 10% African American, 86% percent Caucasian, 2% Hispanic/Latino, 1% Asian and Pacific Islander, and less than 1% American Indian.

With regard to the existing health care system, Allen County has three hospitals—Parkview, Luthern, and St. Joseph of Ft. Wayne. All three are considered tertiary care hospitals by residents of the county (Indiana State Health Department 1994).

There are approximately 73 general practice/family practice physicians, sixteen obstetricians, and eight pediatricians in Allen County. Clinics include Matthew 25 (a clinic that services non-Medicaid, low-income persons of all ages) and Three Rivers Health Services (a clinic which provides full health care services for women and children at one site and WIC services at another site).

Other health care services in Allen County include mental health services for women of reproductive age at fourteen sites; Healthy Families Indiana (child abuse program); Allen County Health Department; and the Regional Administration Office of Children with Special Health Care Services.

St. Joseph County

St. Joseph County is located in north-central Indiana, bordering on Michigan. Population is 247,000, which is 4.4% of Indiana's population. The racial composition is 9.8% African American, 86.9% Caucasian, 2% Hispanic/Latino, 1% Asian and Pacific Islander and .3% American Indian.

With regard to the existing health service system, St. Joseph County has four hospitals: Memorial Hospital, St. Joseph Medical Center, Michiana, and Community Hospital.

There are approximately 95 primary care physicians in St. Joseph County. Additionally, six clinics within the South Bend/Mishawaka area provide primary and preventive care to low-income, Medicaid-insured, and uninsured mothers and children. Other health services include the Healthy Pregnancy and Healthy Babies Free Pregnancy Test Program.

Prenatal care coordination efforts include specialists such as practicing prenatal care coordinators at the Healthy Family Center in Mishawaka, St. Joseph Family Practice Center in South Bend, Veterans Administration in South Bend, and Memorial Hospital Clinic. There are 43 certified care coordinators. Other prenatal care coordination efforts include the St. Joseph County Health Department; it has ten public health nurses who make prenatal and postnatal visits by referrals from physicians, hospitals, and agencies. These public health nurses also provide follow-up visits to children with special needs through referral from Memorial Hospital's intensive care nursery (Indiana State Health Department 1994).

PHASE 1: PREPARING AND ADAPTING TO THE FIELD

The primary aim of this study was to assess the cultural attitude of African Americans concerning the local health care system in two Indiana counties. A secondary objective of the study was to answer one major question, What sociocultural factors (attitudes, beliefs, and values) affect African Americans utilization of prenatal health care services Indiana?

In order to answer this basic question, I was asked to assist a team of public health researchers to investigate this critical health care issue. In collaboration with the Indiana State Health Department Maternal and Child Health division, we developed an innovative research design to investigate not only prenatal health care issues but also cultural, social, historical, political, economic, and public health issues affecting African American populations in Allen and St. Joseph counties.

PHASE 2: MEDICAL ANTHROPOLOGY FIELDWORK TECHNIQUES

To accomplish this applied medical anthropological fieldwork project, a qualitative and quantitative study was developed. Focus groups, individual, in-depth interviews, and surveys were used to collect the cultural attitudinal data as they relate to health care-seeking behavior and prenatal health care issues from residents in both counties.

Overall, this project consisted of four stages: (1) facilitator training sessions, (2) focus group sessions, (3) individual, in-depth interviews, and (4) structured survey questionnaires of African Americans and a control group of Euro-Americans.

In June 1995, I began the facilitator training sessions with local community residents in Ft. Wayne and South Bend. These local community residents were recruited with assistance from the State Health Department.

From July 1995 to September 1995, focus group sessions took place in local community sites in Ft. Wayne and South Bend. Focus group sessions were moderated by facilitators who had participated in the facilitator training sessions. Eleven focus group sessions were held in the two designated sites, five in Ft. Wayne and six in South Bend.

From September 1995 to October 1995, five individual, in-depth interviews were conducted—three in Ft. Wayne and two in South Bend. I conducted 4 of them. Individuals were selected on strictly a volunteer basis. Those who had participated in the focus groups were asked if they would want to volunteer for a more in-depth, one-on-one session.

Finally, from July to September 1995, structured survey questionnaires were distributed to two sets of audiences. All individuals who participated in the focus group sessions were asked to fill out a structured survey questionnaire immediately after each session. Some individuals did, and others decided to fill out the questionnaires at a later date.

The second audience was the control groups of African Americans and Euro-Americans who did not participate in the focus groups. The control groups were sampled at mainstream health care facilities and asked to fill out the structured survey questionnaire. The total number of participants who completed the structured survey questionnaire was as follows:

1. Black Focus Group   =   42
2. Black Control Group =   22
3. Non-Black Control Group = 37

Facilitator Training Sessions

Prior to conducting the focus groups, I trained all the focus group leaders through a facilitator training session held one month prior to the actual focus group sessions. The major purpose of the facilitator training sessions was to ensure reliability and consistency of the number of focus group sessions being conducted in both counties.

There were two facilitator training sessions, one in South Bend and one in Ft. Wayne. These facilitator training sessions occurred one month apart. In each of the training sessions, we encouraged the community volunteers to follow a general guideline for conducting their focus groups. The major objectives that I emphasized in the facilitator training sessions were as follows:

1.   Be flexible.
2.   Learn from your participants.
3.   Be patient.
4.   Guide the discussion.
5.   Remain focused on the topic.
6.   Maintain the structure of the focus group.
7.   Maintain a nonbiased approach.

In the Ft. Wayne facilitator training sessions, five facilitators were present, four women and one man; all facilitators were residents of the local African American community; a pretest of the focus group session occurred one week later; and because of the lack of male facilitators, I became the facilitator in two focus group sessions.

In the South Bend facilitator training sessions, nine facilitators were present, five women and four men; all facilitators were residents of the local African American community; focus group sessions would occur at more neighborhood sites; all facilitators appeared to be well prepared and ready to conduct their individual focus groups; and all facilitiators had established strong networks in the African American community.

For the actual focus group, all potential participants received a letter from the Indiana State Health Department requesting their participation in this study. The local community leaders and the State Health Department made the arrangements as to where and when the focus group sessions would be held in South Bend and Ft. Wayne.

PHASE 3: ETHNOGRAPHIC FIELDWORK DATA ANALYSES

Quantitative Results

The sample size of the black focus and black control groups was 42 and 22 participants, respectively. They differed significantly by gender (p = 0.001) and age category (p = 0.010). Females made up 55.3% and 95.4% of the black focus and black control groups, respectively. The black focus group had a higher percentage of participants 54 years of age and older (31.6% vs.. 4.5%). In contrast, the black control group had a higher percentage of participants between the ages of 13-55 years of age (68.2% vs. 31.6%).

Although not statistically significant, the black focus group compared to the black control group had a higher percentage of participants who were married (35.1% vs. 13.6%), did not have any children (29.7% vs. 9.1%), and reported an approximate average monthly income of $2,001 or more (36.8% vs. 14.3%).

The sample size of the black focus and non-black control groups was 42 and 37 participants, respectively. There were no significant demographic differences between the two groups. However, females made up 55.3% and 76.5% of the black focus and nonblack control groups, respectively. The black focus group had a higher percentage of participants 54 years of age and older (31.6% vs. 14.7%). In contrast, the nonblack control group had a slightly higher percentage of participants between the ages of 13 and 35 years (44.1% vs. 31.6%).

The black focus group compared to the nonblack control group had a higher percentage of participants who were married (35.1% vs. 18.2%), did not have any children (29.7% vs. 9.1%), had 4 or more children (21.6% vs. 11.8%), and reported an approximate average monthly income of $2,001 or more (36.8% vs. 15.1%).

Of the 40 questions asked in the survey, there were two major statistical findings of interest that related to our qualitative cultural themes. For instance, a higher percentage of the black focus group (47.5%) compared to the black control group (27.0%) and the non-black control group (28.5%) would like to choose a doctor or nurse similar to their racial/ethnic background.

In addition, all groups significantly agreed that the county hospital and clinics should have better care for African Americans (black focus group = 89%; black control group = 85%; and nonblack Control group = 73%). This statistical finding indicates a *perceived* problem with the local health systems for African Americans from all the sampled groups.

Qualitative Results

All participants of this study had the opportunity not only to complete the questionnaire but also to write additional comments and provide suggestions. The comments and suggestions varied from one questionnaire to another yet there were a few interesting themes or commonalities of the written responses.

Black Focus Group and Black Control Group Themes

1.   improve health care professional treatment and training;
2.   improve health care accessibility; and
3.   improve national health care system organization.

Theme #1: Improve Health Care Professional Treatment and Training

More care geared toward treating the whole family in addition to specific emergency needs. More doctors and practitioners per population area. Training courses for doctors and nurses in interpersonal and social skills with patients and family members. Need more real listening skills in their training. Most doctors rush you in and out so fast that you wonder if they really hear and understand what you say and feel.

If I could change how a person gets health care treatment, I would design programs and organizations along with proper staffing on educating patient on what type of health care treatment is available, its procedures and purposes for receiving any type of health care treatment. I have heard of too many complaints from patients about improper or inadequate health care and not following or having a daily routine and inadequate staff.

Theme #2: Improve Health Care Accessibility

Increasing access is critical. I do not mean access in terms of number of facilities. Access means not only facilities, but affordability, even for those without the ability to pay themselves. Health care is critical for everyone—haves and have nots. All must make affordability a non-issue when addressing health concerns.

Well for someone like myself who doesn't have a doctor or anything, I think help should be for everyone when it is needed.

Theme #3: Improve the National Health Care System Organization

I would make the health care system more user friendly. The answer to that would be to have some sort of universal health care plan.

I would make it possible for every individual in our country to be able to receive the medical attention needed. If this means keeping monies that are being given to other countries in our own country to take care of our own than so be it. I do believe that every able body should be required to contribute in some way.

Black Focus Group and Non-black Control Group Themes

1.   patient income and accessibility;
2.   patient income and health care professional treatment; and
3.   improve health care professional treatment and training.

Theme #1: Patient Income and Accessibility

Access to care needs to be greatly improved. It is virtually impossible for low-income individuals, especially single males to obtain care for serious but non-critical illnesses if they fall into the no-man's land between major insurance coverage on one hand and medicaid on the other.

That everyone has access to good quality health care, regardless of race or ability to pay; and that everyone would have his/her own personal primary care physician, instead of using the emergency room at a hospital for such a purpose. Also that more preventive care is presented more frequently in the work setting and in the public school system.

Theme #2: Patient Income and Health Care Professional Treatment

There is not equal care; but it's divided along economic lines, not racial ones. Money talks, and the rest walks. Your ability to pay has more to do with your level of care than anything else. If you are without an insurance card, your level of care plummets. I have always believed that money issues or profit in health care is a little extreme. Doctors have bills to pay too. But the entire health care system is out of control. If I could change it, I would guarantee everyone the ability to get the same doctors, care level, and etc ... Right now its really bad out there.

Medicaid patients would be treated with the same respect and care as paying patients. People of poverty and color would have doctors who treat their problems seriously. Doctors should listen to and work with income patients to ensure proper medical health.

Theme #3: Improve Health Care Professional Treatment and Training

Doctors should have patience and hear the person out as to what is bothering them- not ask what you are here for. They are supposed to diagnose what is wrong! I ask where you are hurting at. They should take the time to talk to you and ask what prescriptions you are taking. They should consider all things.

I feel people should help someone who is in need. No matter if it's race or health wise. I have had an African American doctor and he was good at taking care of people. He's warmhearted person and cares about all his patients. As long as you have the heart ... people should be treated equal.

I would hire diverse personnel to work in hospitals, clinics, and doctor's office. People with pleasant attitudes.

The questionnaire themes and comments (extracted from the open-ended section of their questionnaire) from all groups not only highlighted a number of significant issues related to the statistical findings but also provided additional support of the detailed qualitative data collected during the focus group and in-dividual, in-depth interview sessions.

Ft. Wayne Focus Group Themes

In order to provide detailed and in-depth interpretation of the statistical findings, focus groups and individual, in-depth interviews helped to provide clarity and validity to these preliminary statistical findings. There were a total of five focus group sessions in Ft. Wayne from July 20 to August 8, consisting of 15–24 years, 25–54 years, and 55 and older. All the focus group sessions were conducted either by the trained facilitators at community sites in Ft. Wayne and/or by me.

The six major qualitative Ft. Wayne focus group themes were

1. preference for certain health care facilities;
2. type of treatment received;
3. disliked being generalized with certain illnesses;
4. varying degrees of support systems;
5. sought care from African American physicians; and
6. specific generational, social, and cultural lifestyle differences.

Theme #1: Preference for Certain Health Facilities

Qualitative cultural data indicated that a majority of the local African Ameri-can population preferred certain local health care facilities *more* than others primarily because of the past historical relationship with the African American community (positive), the interrelationship of the staff with patients (positive or negative), and the doctor–patient relationship (positive or negative).

Oh yes, my preference is Parkview hospital but I have a new doctor and he only goes to St. Joe. And so I had to see him at St. Joe but my preference is Parkview. Parkview to me, they care more.
Now, I'm just the opposite of her. I have been to St. Joe Hospital several times for heart operations and then back and forth. I always found they were right there for me.

Theme #2: Type of Treatment Received

One of the major reasons how and why African Americans preferred or disliked certain health care professionals was primarily the type of treatment received.

A good doctor is someone that you walk into their office and you tell them what you have been experiencing and they give you dialogue.

I guess I'm a little different because when I go to the doctor I don't know—what's wrong with me, but I know how I feel, you know. The doctor ain't going to sit there and tell me how I feel because I know how I feel. I'm going to tell you how I feel and you figure out what you going to do about it.

Theme #3: Disliked Being Generalized with Certain Illnesses

I've had experiences too. But I will tell you ladies as far as a heart condition, it's a part of—when you go into the hospital and you're a women, even looking as good as you do, a lot of the nurses and doctors in the emergency room will not think that women have heart attacks. Okay? That's been already lined out. My mother has been going through the same thing and she had to go back and forth, back and forth before, you know, she looks good, just like you. They run the EKG, and say there's nothing on the EKG.

So, I would tell this particular doctor, you know, I'm sick, I'm you know, I can't walk to the corner or maybe if I do make it down there I can't make it back home, somebody got to carry me back home or you know, I got to sit there until I feel I'm strong enough to make it back. It gets off into your ethnic questions. Okay? Because of my ethnicity, he said that he felt like I was trying to give him symptoms because I did not want to go back to my job and stay on sick leave.

Theme #4: Varying Degrees of Support Systems

African Americans have varying degrees of support systems that enables individuals to overcome their perceived and/or actual health care barriers in their community.

My mom and dad have been married for—they just had their 23rd anniversary. And I'm the middle out of five kids, and I made the first grandchild. They were real good about it (pregnant) and didn't yell at me or anything. They were good about it.

Because I was scared of what they were going to do. Because when I was younger, I used to be kind of bad. But our family is real close, and so they were kind of upset because I didn't tell them earlier, but they didn't yell at me or nothing. They just said we will work it out.

Theme #5: Sought Care from African American Physicians

A large percentage of African Americans sought care from African American physicians. Although the quality of care and speculation of the physicians' expertise varied from one person to another, local African Americans still preferred African American physicians.

Not really, because I like Dr. A. He's real nice. And him being a pastor has a lot to do with it, I like that. He's real nice, so I would not. I like him. He's a nice doctor. I didn't really have any other choices. He did a real good job. I never had during my pregnancy, I didn't have not one problem. He was real good, and he was a good doctor, and took care of me real well.

I think the average African American in this community goes to the black physicians here. Well, they go, because they are all from Alabama. Everybody is from Alabama. They support all the Alabamians. That is what I have seen here in this particular community. I'm surprised at that, and I'm pleased with it.

Theme # 6: Specific Generational, Social, and Cultural Lifestyle Differences

Each age group experienced specific generational health, social, and cultural lifestyle issues. Often, each age group focused on its own specific health care issues.

They did this to me and I couldn't understand it. I went back and forth and social security said we take $46.90 out of your social security check. Medicaid, they pay the rest. My spin down is $70.00 a month. Right now I pay $24.10, that's what they take out of my social security check, and what I pay is the spin down.

South Bend Focus Group Themes

There were a total of six focus group sessions in South Bend from August 7 to August 10, consisting of age groups 15–24 years, 25–54 years, and 55 years and older. In addition, all the focus group sessions were conducted either by the trained facilitators at community sites in South Bend and/or by me.

The six major themes were as follows:

1.   developed alternative health care practices;

2.   examined preference for certain local health care facilities;
3.   experienced varying degrees of quality care from local
     health care professionals;
4.   disliked being generalized with certain illnesses;
5.   received alternative standards of care from African American
     physicians; and
6.   specific generational health care issues.

Theme #1: Developed Alternative Health Care Practices

African Americans developed alternative health care practices in response to the perceived and/or actual barriers to the local health care system.

I think a lot of the people don't get treatment because historically in most of our families, people just didn't go. You had to be really ill to go to a doctor. And you found other ways. Lots of people practice home remedies and a number of other things that just didn't cause you to go to the doctor. And when you were ill and you got better, you didn't go then.

As a youngster growing up, I only went to the doctor if I was ill. And parents had creative, cultural ways of dealing with illnesses. Like all sorts of teas and all kinds of weird stuff.

I don't know either, but I think that leads to the cultural issues in that, first of all, generally speaking, between African Americans and the medical field there is that mistrust. When somebody says, they don't provide quality service, you surely are not as likely to get us to go there. Just because, historically, we have always tended to listen to Grandmas and their remedies, our great-grandmas and their remedies and such and such. And I think that has something to do with it in terms of this community not seeking out osteopathic care.

Theme #2: Preference for Local Health Care Facilities

Although African Americans have varying attitudes and preferences for local health care facilities, the responses tended to reflect the individual and/or the individual's sociocultural network definition of *quality of care.*
I'd like to say the quality of health care that I've received in St. Joseph County is probably as close to as best in the State of Indiana.

The people there ask the right questions and everything, but I just don't like the way they do it at M_____. It makes me feel inferior or something.

You know what the other thing is? One you see as a public hospital and the other you see as a private. That makes the difference of where you choose to go.

Theme #3: Experienced Varying Degrees of Quality of Care from Local Health Care Professionals

I think the majority of doctors in South Bend are very, very, professional. I believe—I do believe that everything is insurance and money related, which is their job. I mean, they've got to make a living just as well.

I never thought you could tell a doctor what you wanted. But that's what you have to do. You have to assume that responsibility for your ways if you want to get quality care. Otherwise, they'll give you what they have time to give you.

Theme #4: Disliked Being Generalized with Certain Illnesses

A majority of African Americans felt that their diagnosis and/or their prescribed treatment regimen by a local health care professional was primarily based on generalized ethnic health care behavioral assumptions.

But one of my sons went to the emergency room. He ate some peanuts or something. He was allergic to the peanuts sending him into an asthma attack where he couldn't breath so I had to call the emergency ambulance. When they first got to my house they naturally assumed he had been using drugs and that's why he couldn't breathe. But after he got to the hospital emergency room and they began to check him over, they figured out that he was allergic to something and they gave him a shot so he could breathe better. But it   made me mad because they naturally assumed— made an assumption.

On a cultural basis, it may be that they might think your appearance is not up to what they think. You can look in someone's face and just read the disdain that they have for you. They're not really trying to deal with you or that they think you're really interested. Whether it's cultural or economic, it's there, and you think to yourself, well, there's no reason for it. And I'm not sure what it is.

Theme #5: Alternative Standards of Care from African American Physicians

African Americans tended to evaluate, to perceive, and to develop alternative standards of the quality of care from African American physicians than Euro-American physicians.

So we kind of grew up like that, but as we got older and we became teenagers, we went to the black doctors and that was always a pleasant experience. We felt like they liked us. They knew we weren't just somebody coming in there being treated and then they cared about you.

I go to the black doctor first, then I judge them on the type of care that I receive. If I like it then I will stay. If not then I will get another doctor.

I really holistically do not think that sometimes the black doctors are able to go to the updated training stuff. They just don't have the time to go.

My opinion since I've been here for—I won't say how many years—sixty some odd years. I haven't had the problem, because I—because I have dealt with black doctors when I could. Not because he was a black doctor, because he just happened to fit me; and he was good.

Theme #6: Specific Generational Health Care Issues

Each age group among African Americans, particularly the elderly, were very much focused upon their age group's major health care crisis.

You would get tired of it too if every week you had a stack of bills come in. And you get on the phone. You call these toll-free numbers. They put you on a music program or for an hour. And then they come on there, and say—May I help you.

And I therefore think that our government is not fair. I think that there should be something specific set up for senior citizens that's medical, hospitals, medicines, and everything. Because black people do not have the—have like eighty or ninety dollars for one prescription a week.

Well, you know, you hate to act that dumb. But you know, you need to take it to somebody to explain to you why you keep getting all of these bills from Medi-care saying they paid this little portion but they didn't pay this part. And I still owe this much to the doctor. Also as soon you make a visit to the hospital, you start getting all of these letters; and they're so confusing.

Individual, In-Depth Themes

The general purposes of the individual, in-depth profiles were to obtain intimate and detailed knowledge about the individual African American; to gain a comprehensive view of the African American's sociocultural environment and lifestyle; and to generalize from the individual African American to the rest of the local African American population.

There were five individual, in-depth profiles three Fort Wayne residents and two South Bend residents (two women and three men). These individual, in-depth profiles consisted of primarily two age groups: 25–54 years, and 55 years and older. All of these interviews were conducted either by the trained facilitators at Ft. Wayne and South Bend and/or by me.

The six major individual, in-depth profile themes from South Bend and Ft. Wayne were as follows:

1. African Americans' adaptation to local historical health care system issues;
2. African Americans' sociocultural intervention strategies;
3. African Americans' use of alternative medical practices;
4. African Americans' cultural attitudes and preferences for local health care facilities and health care professionals; and
5. African Americans' preference for certain type of physicians.

Theme #1: African American's Adaptation to Local Historical Health Care System Issues

I moved to South Bend at age of six and ... what was much of shock to me were the schools. That's where I learned about segregation. Yet once I understood that from school then I began to look for that in every other place. like in the doctor field. I got a black doctor and I felt kind of comfortable then ... in fact he became our family doctor.

As long as you keep within your boundary lines, you're were okay even today. They sugar-coat it today.

Theme #2: African American Sociocultural Intervention Strategies

Individual African American preferred a variety of new public health and clinical intervention strategies which takes into account more of the social and cultural dynamics of the local African American resident.

My family believes not... that it is better to get checked out. Now with my health care plan and insurance I feel safer now. Even doctors today allow for payment plans... So go to a doctor that is right for you.

African Americans need to become more informed ... about how to take care of ourselves and to get good information and to make good decisions about one's health ... and to study and to know about life in general ... educate ourselves about what we are doing.. and not receiving accept someone else's word.

Theme #3: Use of Alternative Medical Practices

Qualitative cultural data indicated that individual African Americans used and relied upon various traditional preventive home remedies in conjunction with mainstream treatment therapies. The African American preventive health care practices tended to reflect the individual's original place of origin (in the United States), their adaptation to the local social and health care system, and perceived costs of mainstream health care treatment regimens.

Take a teaspoon of honey and drop one lemon drop ... and that would fight the cold. Caster oil would move your bowels to the cold out of your system ... that is if you do not have any money ... this really comes from older generations.

Yes ... especially for colds ... old granddad ... lemon and honey (home remedies). I think we want to ... so we don't have to go to the doctor. Because if we go to the doctor, we are admitting that we can't take care of ourselves. It's false pride sewed into our culture ... particularly black males.

I understand now that the best thing for me to do if I don't know what it is to get to a doctor.

Theme #4: Cultural Attitudes & Preferences for Local Health Care Facilities and Health Care Professionals

Qualitative cultural data indicated that the early experiences with the local social and health issues often times formulated and/or influenced the individual African American's perception of the local health care facilities and health care professionals.

You be surprised what they don't tell the black people today. Like getting help here. Or there... they are not told about these options to help blacks get good health care.

You just won't be treated fairly here. I know very little about the health care field but it's my gut feeling.

Theme #5: Prefer African American Physicians

Qualitative cultural data indicated that the individual African American tended to prefer the African American physicians as their primary doctor primarily because of their early childhood family pattern of seeking care from African American physicians and their perception of commonality due to ethnicity and cultural health beliefs.

There were two black doctors that came here several years ago. They were good ... our family stayed with them for years until they left. The black doctors seemed to be more sensitive to what we need as blacks but after a while your mind believes that they can do more for you than the other doctors.

The development of good network of black doctors... Unite them as one, all health care professionals... And find out what it takes to take care of us.

Reflective Comments

My recommendations to the Indiana State Health Department were as follows:

1. Continual needs assessment of targeted community;
2. Needs assessment of urban and rural communities;
3. Needs assessment of specific subgroups of African Americans;
4. Involvement of local community members with state intervention programs;
5. State collaboration and sponsorship with local outreach programs; and
6. Increase representation of African American health care professionals.

Comments such as the following help to understand why these policy recommendations were important to each county's health care system.

African Americans need to become more informed about how to take care of ourselves and to make good decisions about one's health... and not accept someone else's opinion.

The state should allow minorities in the health care system. I would think there would be funds available for everyone to get into the health field and learn more about the health care field instead of a select few.

CONCLUSION

In view of the public health issues discussed in this pilot study, there is an obvious need to focus on the cultural attitude of African Americans toward the local health care system. Understanding the culture of a population is of special importance in health-related situations because it determines whether a specific population will tend to utilize or avoid available health services. In order to improve the image and perception of the U.S. public health system among all populations, we must continue to merge professional knowledge with community health values and community health needs. Still the issue of *equity* is of major importance to all of us.

POST-EVALUATION QUESTIONS

1. To what degree can the community's perspective of the local health care system affect public health programs?

2. How would you have improved this applied medical anthropological project?

3. To what degree can administrators improve the image of their local public health system?

REFERENCES

Bailey, Eric. 1991. *Urban African American Health Care*. Lanham, MD: University Press of America.
———. 1994a. "The Health Care System and African Americans in Indianapolis." *Journal of the National Medical Association* 86: 11: 853–856. Indiana State Health Department.
———. 1994b. *Impact of SOBRA Expansion on Pregnancy Outcomes in Indiana. Plus Allen, Lake, Marion, St. Joseph, and Vanderburgh Counties*. Briefing Report to the Governor. July.

WEB SITES OF SIGNIFICANCE

National Agency for the Advancement of Colored People

http://www/naacp.org

National Urban League

http://www.nul.org/

Part V

Culture and Health: The Future of African American Health Care Research

Throughout this book, the major focus of each chapter is to highlight the role of culture with today's health care issues. In order for any public health or medical care regimen to be truly effective in the African American community (as well as other ethnic communities), medical anthropologists must develop new cultural health care strategies for specific groups of African Americans. In addition, new cultural health empowerment strategies for public and health professionals are discussed in this part.

Chapter 15

Cultural Health Care Strategies for African Americans

CRITICAL THINKING QUESTIONS

1. What are cultural health strategies?

2. Describe the importance of developing a cultural health strategy for the African American community.

3. How can health care professionals design cultural health strategies for their African American patient population?

INTRODUCTION

Medical anthropology's approach to health care is ideal for any health care researcher, clinician, public health administrator, student, and patient primarily because it is still the one remaining discipline that examines health from a biopsychosociocultural (BPSC) perspective. Biology, psychology, sociology, and culture are all important components to this model.

In this book, however, we have emphasized the *cultural* component of the biopsychosociocultural model due to the fact that there has been less attention to culture and its relationship to health and the difficulty of defining culture as it relates to a particular population. *Culture* is the driving force or essential component to this model.

In order to examine fairly and ethically health care issues associated with the African American population, we must view mortality data, census data, preventive health care data, alternative medical practices data, clinical research data, fieldwork data, and intervention data from a totally different approach. This new approach places *culture* and *cultural relativism* at the forefront of every model that is used to investigate, to treat, or to implement any medical or health care agenda for the African American population.

To reiterate from Chapter 1, *culture* and *cultural relativism* are synonymous terms that are often used together by many scholars and researchers. For example, culture involves the values and belief systems shared by members of a particular group, whereas cultural relativism is an insider's perspective that an outsider should be attempting to obtain when evaluating or examining the values and belief systems of a particular group. Often, however, the health care researcher or clinician views the culture of a group only as a deterrent or barrier to overcome and does not consider obtaining a cultural relativistic perspective of that particular group or patient.

African Americans, for example, are more likely than European Americans to report that during their last visit their physician did not inquire sufficiently about pain, did not tell them how long it would take for prescribed medicine to work, did not explain the seriousness of the illness or injury, and did not discuss tests or examination findings. Fewer than three-fifths of African Americans were completely satisfied with the care provided during their last hospitalization, compared with over three-fourths of European Americans (Blendon et al. 1989).

Despite such trends that indicate a lack of effort in cultural relativism from health care providers, a number of clinical and community-based programs have achieved varying degrees of cultural relativism. The following sections highlight selected cultural relativistic clinical and community health programs that have attempted to introduce culture into the model of intervention. In addition, this part focuses upon cultural relativistic approaches of health care to specific age, gender, and socioeconomic segments of the African American population.

CULTURE AND AFRICAN AMERICAN ELDERLY

African American elders are a diverse group, and it is important to recognize this group's heterogeneity (Brangman 1995). No typical African American elder exists. They can vary from an elder living in the rural South to an elder in an urban area in the Northeast (Brangman). Brangman states that they may have been born in the northern or southern parts of the United States or be members of a subgroup, as are immigrants from various parts of the Caribbean, such as Jamaica or Haiti. Their history, religious, educational, socioeconomic, and marital statuses, and cultural backgrounds must be taken as a starting point for understanding the individual, while avoiding overgeneralizations and stereotypes (Brangman 1995: 16; Mouton, Johnson, and Cole 1995).

Martin and Panicucci's (1996) study of 40 elderly African American women's health behaviors and beliefs highlighted the difference in this study's results versus stereotypical beliefs associated with elderly African American women. Findings revealed that southern, community-living African American older women generally have a high level of adherence to commonly recommended health promotion/disease prevention habits.

Martin and Panicucci stipulated that a most likely explanation for the high levels of adherence may stem from their cultural and religious doctrines that discourage certain unhealthy practices such as excessive alcohol consumption, cigarette smoking, and ineffective coping outlets. Because study findings indicate that African American older women want to maintain their health, increased attention must be directed to the importance of primary prevention behaviors as an assertion of control over one's future health, well being, and quality of life (Martin and Panicucci 1996: 47).

Martin and Panicucci (1996) suggested that nurses must set into place interventions that enhance the perceptions of relevance regarding the lifestyle practice of regular exercise. Regular community-based exercise classes in churches, residential settings, senior centers, or other frequently attended community sites would increase the likelihood of regular participation in exercise (47).

Finally, it is clear that more and more African Americans are living longer and are in better health. It is imperative that health care administrators develop and plan culturally sensitive health care services for older African Americans from various social and cultural backgrounds.

CULTURE AND AFRICAN AMERICAN WOMEN

In recent years, there have been a new consciousness and awareness concerning women's health within the biomedical and health care community (Pinn 1995). In 1990, the National Institutes of Health (NIH) established the Office of Research on Women's Health for the purpose of strengthening and developing research initiatives for women in all communities. In fact, one of NIH's specific initiatives in 1995 focused upon researcher behavioral and cultural factors related to women and disease prevention/intervention (Pinn 1995: 10).

One particular large-scale study that has developed from this research initiative on women's health is the Black Women's Health Study. Funded by the National Cancer Institute and conducted by a team of epidemiologists from Boston and Howard Universities, the Black Women's Health Study is the largest epidemiological study of African American women yet conducted (Rosenberg, Adams-Campbell and Palmer 1995). This study expects to find answers concerning issues of obesity and diseases; relation of physical activity to cardiovascular disease, diabetes mellitus, and breast cancer; and the relation of cigarette smoking to cardiovascular disease (Rosenberg, Adams-Campbell, and Palmer 1995). Moreover, the answers to these health issues will provide some general insight into the cultural health-seeking pattern among African American women.

Yet there still remains a gap of information concerning how culture influences health practices among African American women (Mouton et al. 1997). Kathleen Jennings (1996), a nurse practitioner, has identified a number of social and cultural factors that have influenced African American women to not participate in cancer-related health promotion programs:

1. cancer as a death sentence;
2. spirituality and cancer among blacks;
3. negative attitudes regarding cancer screening and treatment among African Americans;
4. distrust of the health care system;
5. exclusion of blacks and females from health care research;
6. exclusion of African Americans from community-based screening programs; and
7. barriers and social stigmas experienced by African American women. (56)

Despite these social and cultural barriers, Jennings highlighted six cultural relativistic intervention strategies that nurse practitioners should use when working with African American women. They are described as follows:

1. Appreciate: relating sister to sister.
2. Negotiate: creating community kinship.
3. Integrate: combining health beliefs and health behaviors.
4. Educate: empowering women through knowledge.
5. Advocate: "I've got your back" (explained later).
6. EVALUATE: application of the nursing process. (57)

For example, relating sister to sister implies that the nurse practitioner must develop "sister circles" within African American communities for the purpose of influencing cancer health behaviors (57). In order to develop these "sister circles," Jennings suggests that nurse practitioners must (1) develop an understanding of the African American culture, its issues, its values, and its health concerns; (2) seek out the formal sister circles in the community; (3) be visible in places where women meet; and (4) identify and respect the reverent power of community leaders.

Second, Jennings suggests that empowering women through knowledge means the following:

1. Screening programs should be designed to give accurate information, not just provide an examination;
2. Educational programs should address the psychosocial issues of being black and female;
3. Educational programs should be user-friendly; and
4. Educational programs should provide information regarding community resources available for clients to access. These types of educational strategies will truly empower women with the knowledge to change health behaviors.

Finally, Jennings suggests that "I've got your back," referring to being committed to support someone in need, is an important concept in the African American community. Nurse practitioners must be committed in the fight against cancer in order to win the trust of the community and to create a perception of a caring attitude (57).

In summary, although the health care field has awakened to the specific health issues concerning African American women, there still remains a lack of information and understanding on how cultural factors influence health behavior. The use of small focus group sessions with African American women will provide answers to a number of health issues affecting African American women's health. The urgency for a cultural relativistic perspective as it relates to African American women's health is desperately needed.

CULTURE AND AFRICAN AMERICAN MEN

Year after year, the health data associated with African American men continue to show strikingly large disparity of health outcomes when compared to other segments of the U.S. population. Yet when viewed separately, African American men have showed improved health outcomes in such areas as life expectancy, heart disease mortality, stroke mortality, lung cancer mortality, and unintentional injury mortality (U.S. Department of Health & Human Services 1994).

As for African American women, research on the relationship between culture and health practices among African American men has been very minimal or very generalized. One area of research that has focused specifically among African American men is prostate cancer.

Prostate cancer originates in the prostate gland, a male genital gland about the size of a walnut that is located in front of the rectum, behind the base of the penis, and under the bladder. Because of its location, a physician can directly examine the part of the gland where most tumors occur (American Cancer Society 1998: 1).

Prostate cancer is the most commonly diagnosed form of nondermatologic cancer among men in the United States and is second only to lung cancer as a cause of cancer-related death (American Cancer Society 1998). At all ages, African American men tend to be diagnosed with the disease at later stages and to die of prostate cancer more often than European American men do (American Cancer Society 1998). Lack of cancer awareness has been identified as a cause of poor survival and increased mortality rates among African American men (Collins 1997; Demark-Wahnefried 1995).

One particular study interested in the African American adult males' knowledge and perceptions of prostate cancer found that cultural health beliefs influenced health care seeking (Price et al. 1993). The results from 290 randomly selected African American men living in the seven largest cities in Ohio (Columbus, Cincinnati, Cleveland, Toledo, Dayton, Akron, and Canton) revealed that a majority of men did not perceive themselves as susceptible to prostate cancer. Additionally, 45% percent of the men perceived prostate cancer as a death sentence, and another 28% were not sure if it would kill them (Price et al. 1993: 945). Price et al. stated that when you add to this perception the fact that one in five men claimed that the cost of a prostate examination would be a significant barrier to having their prostates examined, you have a condition that helps explain why so many African American males have prostate cancer diagnosed at advanced stages.

With regard to prostate cancer intervention, Price et al. suggest that health educators must realize that unless they oversell the importance of their interventions, they may create a problem of "victim blaming." In other words, some health educators may believe that African American males do not engage in preventive behaviors only because they are ignorant of their risks and the signs and symptoms of prostate cancer (946). Price et al. contend that not only does this type of thinking fail to appreciate how health behaviors develop and are sustained but also a major portion of the higher prostate cancer mortality rate in African American males is related to socioeconomic inequities, and discrimination and its relation to lack of access to health care.

In conclusion, Price et al. (1993) and Powell et al. (1997) suggest that there is a need for increased public education directed specifically at African American males. Cultural relativistic education intervention should be directed toward symptom recognition and more realistic assessments of the benefits of regular prostate cancer examinations (Price et al. 1993: 947). Moreover, clinicians who have direct cultural experiences with African American men can help focus specific education interventions and research efforts that provide relevant information to develop appropriate prostate cancer initiatives for specific populations of African American men (Guidry et al. 1998; Weinrich et al. 1998; and Meyers et al. 1994).

CULTURE AND AFRICAN AMERICAN ADOLESCENT FEMALES

Adolescence is a period of significant life transition, during which children cross the bridge into adulthood (Adams et al. 1995). Behaviors established during this period are often carried into adult life. Adams et al. (1995) state that health behaviors established prior to adulthood can significantly influence health and longevity, both in the short term and later in life.

In 1992, the Centers for Disease Control and Prevention conducted the National Health Interview Survey–Youth Risk Behavior Survey (NHIS-YRBS). The NHIS–YRBS was a collaborative effort of the Division of Health Interview Statistics, the National Center for Health Statistics, and the Division of Adolescent and School Health of the National Center for Chronic Disease Prevention and Health Promotion. Of the 13,789 youth identified as eligible for the NHIS-YRBS, 10,645 completed questionnaires, representing an estimated 77.2% of eligible respondents (Adams et al. 1995).

With regard to weight control, youths 12–21 years of age were asked questions to measure weight control practices that included perceived weight, what, if anything, they were trying to do about their weight, attempts in the past week to lose or keep from gaining weight, and type of weight control attempts in past week (Adams et al. 1995: 15). Adams et al. found that African American adolescent females (36%) were less likely than European American adolescent females (46.1%) to perceive themselves as being overweight. In addition, African American female teens (41.5%) were less likely than European American females (59.5%) and Hispanic females (55.1%) to report any attempt to lose or keep from gaining weight in the past week. Overall, the data show that proportionately, fewer African American female and male youths considered themselves overweight compared with European American female and male youths.

The importance of these national health data on the perceptions of weight control among African American adolescent females relates to the issue of obesity and its health consequences. Obesity rates among African American women are significantly higher than rates for European American women (Kumanyika 1994). Moreover, chronic disease profiles of minority populations indicate that African Americans have higher than average cardiovascular disease-related mortality (Kumanyika 1990; Levinson et al. 1985; and Otten et al. 1990). These health trends and mortality suggest an urgent need for obesity prevention programs for African American adolescent females.

To determine whether obesity prevention programs could work effectively in the African American community, Stolley and Fitzgibbon (1997) designed a culturally specific obesity prevention for low-income, African American adolescent females and their mothers who live in Chicago's inner city. Using the information gathered in a pilot project, Stolley and Fitzgibbon developed a curriculum that addressed the particular cultural and social needs of this population.

First, Stolley and Fitzgibbon felt that parental participation with this population was imperative given the mothers' limited access to dietary and physical activity information, their need for nutrition and health knowledge, and their need for support in making dietary changes. Second, the program was held at a local tutoring program. Third, all activities involving tasting foods, comparing high-fat to low-fat foods, changing recipes, and planning meals were done with foods identified in 24-hour recalls gathered in the pilot project. In addition, subjects in this program were asked to bring in their favorite recipes or foods to be analyzed for fat and caloric content. Fourth, attention to the availability of certain products was given in classes addressing menu planning. Fifth, culturally relevant music and dance were used for a number of exercise and diet-related activities. Finally, appropriate materials gathered from magazines geared toward African Americans were distributed and reviewed for important information on diet and exercise (155).

Stolley and Fitzgibbon found that over the course of a twelve–week program treatment, mothers exhibited a significant decrease in saturated fat and dietary fat, coupled with an increase in parental support. Following the intervention, the mothers who participated in the program reported receiving less than 32% of their calories from fat and an average intake of 11.5 grams of saturated fat, compared to a pretreatment diet of 40% daily calories from fat and nearly 14 grams of saturated fat (159). Stolley and Fitzgibbon stated that the intervention had a positive effect on mothers' level of support and role modeling of healthy eating behavior for their daughters.

The treatment daughters reported only minor changes in their percentage of calories from fat at posttreatment. Although daughters' behaviors changed only minimally during the twelve-week intervention, Stolley and Fitzgibbon contend that the mothers' modeling behaviors will change the daughters' behaviors in time. Follow-up data will offer insight regarding this issue (159).

Along with parental participation, Stolley and Fitzgibbon believed that other components were imperative to the success of the program. These cultural relativistic components included

1. conducting the program in a safe and familiar community location;
2. incorporation of culturally appropriate music, dance, and media;
3. acknowledgment and knowledge of neighborhood markets in which families shop;
4. acknowledgment and inclusion of foods commonly prepared and eaten by families as identified through 24-hour recalls; and
5. attention to the challenges of adopting a low-fat dietary plan within a strict financial budget (163).

Other factors that Stolley and Fitzgibbon (1997) believe could enhance the effectiveness of the program include (1) a longer-term intervention, (2) follow-up booster sessions to support maintenance of dietary changes, (3) inclusion of a more intensive exercise component, and (4) spending class time on actual preparation of low-fat meals.

In conclusion, this obesity prevention program for African American adolescent females attempted not only to work within the social and cultural parameters of this particular African American population but also to challenge many of the cultural dietary eating patterns of African American adolescent females and their mothers (Walcott-McQuigg 1995). This cultural relativistic approach to dietary intervention and weight control for African American adolescent females provides a framework for understanding how cultural and social factors influence positive health behavioral patterns.

CULTURE AND AFRICAN AMERICAN ADOLESCENT MALES

Much of what has been written and researched about African American adolescent males' health and social behavioral outcomes has been negative and downright gloomy. The health and social data that are often cited in the literature and reported in the media are the homicide rate and sexually transmitted diseases.

According to the National Center for Health Statistics (1995), the homicide rates for black males (72.5 per 100,00) were eight times higher than for white males (9.4 per 100,000) and nearly five times higher than for black females (13.9 per 100,000) as for white females (3.0 per 100,000). Among African

American youth, the homicide rate (77.9 per 100,000) was eight to nine times those for European American (9.6) and Asian American youths (8.8) (NCHS 1994: 29). The cause for this disparity in homicide rates is multifacteted—in other words factors such as personal situational issues, societal discrimination, cultural historical racism, persistent unemployment, peer pressure, and lack of formal education all contribute to the high rate of homicide among African American adolescent males.

With regard to African American male sexual behavior and the risk for HIV infection, the cause for the high prevalence rate of HIV infection is also multi-facteted. Whitehead (1997), for example, found that broader historical and so-ciocultural issues associated with African American adolescent males and mid-dle-aged men contributed to the disproportionately high rate of HIV infection.

Between the fall of 1989 and the spring of 1992, members of the Cultural Systems Analysis Group (CuSAG) conducted eight AIDS-related qualitative research projects in Baltimore, other Maryland locations, and Washington, D.C.. Through open-ended, group, and ethnographic interviews and full neighborhood ethnographies, Whitehead (1996) and CuSAG members interviewed more than 600 men and women in these studies. The data reported in this study derived primarily from interviews with more than 350 males.

The sample consisted of males ranging in age from 10 to 49 years, with most falling between 14 and 29 years. Whitehead (1996) and the CuSAG members recruited males with the assistance of research assistants who resided in the study neighborhoods, from community-based organizations, health departments and other public agencies, and STD and pediatric clinic, and through network "snowball" techniques.

The qualitative analyses from the interviews highlighted several themes. One theme in particular was referred to as *male gender fragmentation*. Whitehead (1996) stipulated that we need to explore male gender fragmentation as a risk factor of HIV transmission in low-income communities. According to White-head, adolescent African American males need a masculinity transformation primarily because the existing constructs of ideal masculinity are conducive to a fragmented masculinity. In other words, the process of becoming a male in our gender-biased society is incorrect. Our society teaches young males inappropri-ate ways of achieving adulthood.

The goal of masculinity transformation is to achieve a sense of masculine gender identity as a whole (436). Masculine transformation is a strategy of empowerment that moves away from notions of masculinity that focus on gain-ing economic capacity to achieve sexual control or on sexual power to achieve social (with male peers) or economic status. Furthermore, Whitehead stated that masculine transformation emphasizes community service, goal-setting, and dis-cipline in achieving goals and integrates body, mind, and spirit.

The cultural relativistic strategy resulting from Whitehead's masculine trans-formation involves peer training in which older, more mature males, including low-income males, work with preadolescent and adolescent boys and young adult men. It helps men on their road to masculine wholeness and works to help younger men overcome their fragmented masculinity (437). Thus, Whitehead recommends masculine transformation, along with the usual HIV/AIDS materials, to effectively address HIV/AIDS among African American adolescent males in low-income American communities.

CULTURE AND CLINICAL TRIAL RESEARCH STUDIES

Most clinical encounters can be analyzed as an interaction between two cultures—the culture of "medicine" and the culture of "patients" (Pachter 1994: 690). Pachter states that these two groups often have different perceptions, attitudes, knowledge, communicative styles, and approaches toward health-related issues. Individuals from each group think about health and illness from different perspectives (Pachter 1994: 690; Toliver-Weddington 1990).

For many African Americans, a visit with their physician tends to be a challenging encounter primarily because each has a different approach to the diagnosis of an illness and the procedure for treatment. The difficulties many African Americans have had with clinicians can best be illustrated by studying attitudinal beliefs among African Americans participating in clinical trials.

To compare attitudes toward participation in cancer clinical trials, Mouton et al. (1997) conducted a cancer clinical trial among African American and European American women. Of the 80 women surveyed, the average age was 62 years (range: 37 to 86 years). Fifty-one (63.3%) were European American, and 29 (36.8%) were African American (723).

Mouton et al. found the following:

1. Almost one-third (32.1%) of the African American women agreed or strongly agreed that scientists cannot be trusted compared with only 4.1% of European Americans (p = .001) who believed this.
2. Twenty-eight percent (28.6%) of the African American women agreed or strongly agreed that researchers did not care about them, while only 13.7% of European American women chose this response.
3. Thirty-seven percent of African American women compared with 2% of European American women preferred to be treated by an African American scientist (p = .014).

In general, African American women felt that clinical research was unethical, that researchers did not care about them, and that by participating in research, they would not have access to better care (726). This study corroborates the findings of Harris et al. (1996) and Freedman (1998) that African Americans fear clinical trials and feel a lack of trust from the medical system.

Mouton et al. (1997) suggest that their findings also support the possibility that a major impediment for African American participation in clinical research is a lack of trust. This lack of trust is precisely the cultural factor that needs to be addressed by clinical researchers and clinicians.

In fact, Mouton et al. addressed this "lack of trust" cultural attitude among African Americans and suggested three major strategies. First, to overcome the barrier of distrust, investigators could include influential community members in the planning stages of clinical trial recruitment, as the community leaders might help dispel some of the suspicion held by the African American community. Second, inclusion of African American investigators in leadership roles also can help alleviate some of the mistrust in the community. Third and perhaps most importantly, facilitating institutional changes in a cultural relativistic manner that promotes the provision of needed health services for the African American community can promote a better working relationship for future research (727).

Finally, clinical researchers must undergo cultural relativistic training, that is, training that includes a much better cultural appreciation of the group being studied. The history, customs, folk beliefs, and values of a people are particularly important to recognize. Often, clinical researchers are devoid of an understanding, appreciation, and ethical responsibility to the people whom they study. African Americans are very sensitive and astute to these feelings. That is why the African American community continues to avoid clinical trials and to feel the mistrust from the medical system. Opening the lines of communication around this issue can lead to an alliance between African Americans, clinical researchers, and clinicians (Pachter 1994).

CULTURE AND PUBLIC HEALTH INTERVENTION PROGRAMS

Public health intervention screening programs were originally designed (1) to stimulate change in family and community knowledge and behavior relating to the prevention of disease; (2) to inform about the use of available health resources; and (3) to improve the environmental, economic, and educational factors related to health (Geiger 1972). Since their inception during the 1960s and 1970s, however, public health intervention screening programs have primarily used conventional approaches to health improvement. That is, the need is not merely for prevention and curative health services or the distribution of services to passive recipients but also for the active involvement of local populations in ways that preserve or repattern their knowledge, attitudes, and motivation concerning major health care issues. Thus, when health care professionals design a culturally relativistic public health screening program, it is intended to address five major issues:

1. to alert a target group to health issues,
2. to help them make choices,
3. to maintain some of their traditional health care practices,
4. to encourage them to try new health care practices, and
5. to inform them of the most straight forward and effective behavioral alternatives for health promotion. (Bailey 1991: 1269)

For instance, Chapter 10 provided an example of a culturally relativistic and culturally competent public health intervention. Bailey's (1991) study as well as many others (Braithwaite and Taylor 1994; Whitehead 1996; Voorhees et al. 1996) show that culturally oriented public health intervention programs have been very successful in reaching the African American community.

Two types of programs, in particular, have been recognized for their culturally relativistic approach to public health intervention for the African American community. First, there are the cancer intervention programs that use cultural institutions and cultural networks associated with African Americans for program implementation and effectiveness. Second, there is the use of the ethnographic approach to gather cultural health data associated with African Americans for the purpose of empowering the community. A brief discussion of these two types of programs should provide the reader with the understanding, insight, and strategy as to the reasons that the cultural relativistic approach to health care is so important.

Recently, cancer prevention programs have developed alternative strategies in reaching their target populations (Yancey and Walden 1994; Mandelblatt et al. 1993; Suarez et al. 1993 and 1994; Tatum et al. 1997; Curry et al. 1994; and Michielutte et al. 1989). Interestingly, the programs that have been most effective are the ones implementing a cultural relativistic approach. For example, Erwin et al. (1992) as well as some local African American women developed an outreach breast and cervical cancer education program specifically for African American women called the Witness Project.

The Witness Project was designed to increase the number of women who practice regular cancer screening through breast self-examination (BSE), mammography, clinical breast examination (CBE), pelvic exam, and Pap tests. At the heart of the Witness Project are African American women who talk to other women about the importance of early detection of cancer—either as witness role models (WRMs) or lay health advisers (LHAs) (Witness Project 1998: 4). The Witness programs are presented in the African American community through local churches or other cultural institutions.

Erwin, Spatz, and Turturro (1992) stated that the intended effort of the Witness Project was to empower others to take responsibility for their health and to practice early detection behaviors. Specifically, the role models challenge the excuses women use for not performing BSE or having mammograms (313). Furthermore, Erwin, Spatz, and Turturro emphasized that direct educational methods are the most effective means of communication in African American populations, particularly when the person making the contact is culturally and socioeconomically similar.

Overall, the Witness Project is a starting point for changing the behavior of African American women with regard to BSE and mammograms. Erwin, Spatz, and Turturro stated that the first step is awareness and prioritization within the community of African American women to address the issues and risk of breast cancer.

Another cultural relativistic cancer prevention program involves the use of beauty salons as an avenue of reaching African American women. Forte (1995) stated that African American women have evolved a unique oral cultural tradition around the beauty salons. This oral exchange of family histories and information remains important to the preservation of African American culture and social interaction. African American women, including those 50 and older, regularly network, exchange information, and talk about local news and issues in beauty salons, and beauticians are often opinion leaders within this community (180).

Using the beauty salons as a cultural focal point, Forte conducted outreach breast cancer screening awareness programs in underserved communities in Los Angeles. Although there are no current outcome data to determine their effectiveness, Forte contends that beauty salons are an ideal place for community-based breast cancer intervention programs to begin. Since African American beauty salons are 90% African American, breast cancer outreach intervention would work well in this setting. In effect, these are precisely the cultural institutions that are often overlooked when public health administrators and health care researchers plan to conduct a community outreach program for African American women.

Finally, the third cultural relativistic approach to cancer prevention that deserves mention in this section is the Forsyth County Cancer Screening (FoCaS) Project. Funded by the National Cancer Institute as one of six Public Health Approaches to Breast and Cervical Cancer Screening grants, the FoCaS Project was designed to test the effectiveness of clinical inreach and community outreach interventions to improve screening utilization by low-income, minority women in rural and urban areas (Tatum et al. 1997: 43).

Tatum et al. (1997) state that the major objectives of the FoCaS Project were to reduce the burden of breast and cervical cancer by improving knowledge, attitudes, and participation in breast and cervical cancer screening and to identify barriers to early cancer detection faced by the target population and health care providers. Secondary objectives were to assess and improve compliance with follow-up recommendations for abnormal findings from mammography, clinical breast examinations, and Pap tests through an inreach program at Reynolds Health Center (RHC) (43).

The FoCaS Project was conducted in four phases over a four-year period. Tatum et al. (1997) described the project as follows:

1. Phase One—protocols were finalized and providers from Reynolds Health Center and other health facilities that served the target population were surveyed. Women in the housing communities were also surveyed regarding cancer screening knowledge, attitudes, and practices. A Community Advisory Board for Forsyth County was also formed in the first year of the project.
2. Phase Two—the inreach (clinic-based) and outreach (community-based) interventions for promoting screening and follow-up of abnormalities were implemented.
3. Phase Three—a follow-up survey of women and providers.
4. Phase Four—the transfer of successful interventions to the comparison communities. (44)

The key components to the FoCaS Project were the selection of the Advisory Board and the community analysis. In particular, the community analysis helped to guide the direction of the intervention.

Tatum et al. (1997) stated that their community analysis consisted of a structured process that began with a careful investigation of the target population and observing the daily lives of the residents and progressed through a systematic review of vital statistics of the community, the local health care delivery system, social and physical environment, communication networks, and social organization. In addition, interviews with key community residents and focus groups with community residents helped to provide the community analysis with the type of cultural awareness and understanding of the framework that the health education programs needed to utilize (45).

The results of this cultural relativistic approach to cancer prevention were the development of five approaches to cancer intervention. The five approaches included utilization of mass media, the continuation of community classes to teach about breast and cervical cancer prevention and control, a focus on the high degree of religiosity of the women, utilization of information centers to distribute printed materials at "points of sale" near each housing community and in the housing communities, and a community-wide cancer awareness event (46). Three of the five approaches were particularly culturally relativistic.

First, community education classes were held regularly in each of the housing communities. The classes were structured to provide participatory learning and were conducted in a relaxed, nonthreatening atmosphere in the housing communities (47). Second, to demonstrate and explain God's role in good health, an inspirational segment "Healthy Spirit" was included in each community class. Additionally, an outreach church intervention program entitled, "Taking Care of Our Sisters" was developed. Third, a day long outdoor festival called "Women Fest" was a community cancer education event presented in a positive atmosphere (47–48).

Although the long-term assessment of the FoCaS Project has not yet been determined, Tatum et al. suggested that when considering alternative routes for reaching the African American population, a constant evaluation of the status of the community is required. What was apparent early in the design of this project was that the status of this population was ever changing, and successful outreach intervention strategies were updated constantly (49). Overall, several types of intervention strategies were utilized to communicate information, address barriers, and improve participation rates for breast and cervical cancer screenings.

CULTURE AND HEALTHY PEOPLE 2010

Healthy People is the prevention agenda for the Nation. It is a statement of national opportunities--a tool that identifies the most significant preventable threats to health and focuses public and private sector efforts to address those threats (*Healthy People 2010* Fact Sheet 1998). *Healthy People 2000*, which was released in 1990, is a comprehensive agenda with 319 objectives organized into 22 priority areas. The overarching goals are to increase years of healthy life, reduce disparities in health among different population groups, and achieve access to preventive health services.

Healthy People 2010 will address similar topics as *Healthy People 2000* but also highlight such emerging issues such as changing demographics, advances in preventive therapies, and new technologies (*Healthy People 2010* Fact Sheet 1998). One area of emphasis for *Healthy People 2010* is effective community health promotion for the twenty-first century.

Healthy People 2010 states that for community health programs to be truly effective in the future, they must strive to do the following:

1. Involve members of the populations served and their gate keepers in the community assessment and planning process;
2. Be culturally competent, age-appropriate, and gender-specific;
3. Must be supported by accurate, appropriate, and accessible information derived from a prevention science base; and
4. Ensure that results are appropriate and that the content and the prevention efforts developed are tailored to meet the needs of the communities and populations being served. (*Healthy People 2010* Fact Sheet 1998: 7)

These four strategies are significant to *Healthy People 2010* primarily because, currently barriers that deter some people from accessing appropriate health services and health promotion programs and because many health programs are not designed with sensitivity to the diverse health beliefs, practices, use patterns, and attitudes of the many ethnic, cultural, gender, and age groups living in America today.

It becomes quite apparent that in order to accomplish the community health objectives for *Healthy People 2010*, a cultural relativistic and medical anthropological approach is a necessity for all those who work in the health care and public health fields. As Braithwaite and Lythcott (1989) stated, "because health behaviors are culture-bound, primary prevention efforts that address preventable disease and illness must emerge from a knowledge of and a respect for the culture of the target community to ensure that both the community organization and development effort and any intervention that emerge are culturally sensitive and linguistically appropriate" (283).

CULTURE AND CULTURAL HEALTH EMPOWERMENT
STRATEGIES FOR THE PUBLIC AND HEALTH PROFESSIONALS

Throughout this book, we have attempted to show how culture is connected to health. African Americans are a unique and diverse group of people. Although similar experiences are threaded within their lifestyle and cultural makeup such as spirituality, family and social networks, and lay health care systems, individuals and families should be assessed for their own unique perceptions of their health needs and for cultural factors that influence how health problems will be managed or prevented (Russell and Jewell 1992: 168).

One of the keys in connecting African American culture with health issues has to do with the concept of empowerment. Empowerment is a process of increasing control by individuals/groups over consequences that are important to the individual/group and to others in the broader community (Braithwaite and Lythcott 1989; and Fawcett et al. 1982). In other words, African Americans need to find ways to take charge of their health.

Culture—the individual's health belief system and the individual's cultural health patterns—is connected to the individual's health status. One approach that can assist individual African Americans is using culture (values, beliefs, and patterns) to ascertain the type of response and/or care that they want and deserve. By placing culture within the concept of empowerment, individuals can be helped to make positive health decisions they understand within their belief system. The following are cultural health empowerment strategies for cultural groups such as (1) the African American patient; (2) the African American community activist; (3) the African American health care professional; (4) the non-African American health care professional; (5) the African American public health administrator; (6) the non-African American public health administrator; (7) the African American health care researcher; and (8) the non-African American health care researcher.

African American Patient

Here are five cultural health empowerment strategies for the African American patient:

1. Make a list of all the "healthy" things that you do for yourself.
2. Make a list of all the "non-healthy" things that you do to yourself.
3. Select from the "healthy" and "nonhealthy" list your most favorite items.
4. Share your selections with your close family members, significant other, health care provider, and/or spiritual leader and then decide whether you should continue your "healthy" and "nonhealthy" activities in the context of a minor or major illness.
5. If you are unsure or not satisfied with your consultation, seek additional information from another familial/caregiving network person and/or health care provider.

The primary purpose of this cultural health empowerment strategy takes into account African Americans' cultural health beliefs and cultural health network, thereby making the decision in seeking care easier and more comfortable for the African American patient.

African American Community Activist

Here are five cultural health empowerment strategies for the African American community activist:

1. Make a list of all the health and social problems in your community.
2. Using the applied medical anthropological strategies for conducting research, interview members of your community and determine what they perceive as the most significant health and social problems of your community.
3. Select the health and social problems that are priorities to you and the information gathered from the community residents.
4. Share this information with other community activists in your neighborhood.
5. Formulate a new health and social community-based organization that can obtain funding to address the health and social problems in your community.

The primary purpose of this cultural health empowerment strategy takes advantage of the cultural network already established by the community activists, gives them an organization that truly represents the community, and provides them a constructive opportunity to change the health and social problems within their community.

African American Health Care Professional

Here are the five cultural health empowerment strategies for the African American health care professional:

(1) Perceive each patient as a part of your extended family (Post and Weddington 1997).
(2) Encourage open dialogue with your patient and their family members during time of visit and follow-up with a phone call/card at their place of residence.
(3) Explain thoroughly your diagnosis, prognosis, and treatment suggestions to the patient and a close family/friend of the patient and listen closely to their response.
(4) Seek a support system with other African American health care professionals and share your strategies with less-experienced colleagues.
(5) Establish a strong community connection with an African American cultural institution such as a church, community-based organization or non-profit organization.

The primary purpose of this cultural health empowerment strategy is to maintain the cultural connection that African American health care professionals have with their community and to broaden the model of disease and treatment regimen for the African American patient.

The Non-African American Health Care Professional

Here are five cultural health empowerment strategies for the non-African American health care professional. These strategies are for those who have had little or limited exposure to the African American patient.

1. Encourage open dialogue with your patient and family members during the time of visit and follow-up with a phone call/card at their place of residence.
2. Listen closely and maintain a comfortable, relaxed presence in your interaction with the patient and the family/friend.
3. Explain thoroughly your diagnosis, prognosis, and treatment suggestions to the patient and a close family/friend.
4. Seek the advice of an African American health care professional to deal more effectively with the health and lifestyle issues of your African American patients (Johnson et al. 1996).
5. Volunteer your time with local community health screening programs.

The primary purpose of this cultural health empowerment strategy is to show to African American patients and their family your sincerity in understanding and connecting with them and to show to other African American health care professionals that you are attempting to become connected to the larger extended network of the African American community.

The African American Public Health Administrator

Here are five cultural health empowerment strategies for the African American public health administrator:

1. Collate all the health, social, and epidemiological data associated with your public health initiative for the community.
2. Using the applied medical anthropological strategies for conducting research, interview key community leaders and community residents and determine how your public health initiative can fit within their priorities.
3. Show that your public health initiative is related to other health initiatives primarily because health issues are all interrelated, and each issue helps to establish the overall well-being of the community.
4. Use your individual and/or familial connections to the cultural institutions within the African American community and begin to market your new public health initiative.

5. Explain thoroughly the priorities, the budget, and the politics of your public health initiative to the community.

The primary purpose of this cultural health empowerment strategy is to combine the documented public health data with the cultural health data from the African American community for the purpose of developing a public health initiative that the community actually needs.

The Non-African American Public Health Administrator

Here are five cultural health empowerment strategies for the non-African American public health administrator. These strategies are for those who have had little or limited exposure to the African American community.

1. Collate all the health, social, and epidemiological data associated with your public health initiative for the African American community.
2. Attempt to not generalize these findings to the entire local African American population.
3. Using the applied medical anthropological strategies for conducting research, interview key community leaders and community residents and determine how your public health initiative can fit within their priorities.
4. Seek the advice of and include, an African American or non-African American public health administrator who has worked extensively with the African American community at large and who has developed a good working relationship with the African American communities.
5. Explain thoroughly the priorities, the budget, and the politics of your public health initiative to the African American community.

The primary purpose of this cultural health empowerment strategy is to give the non-African American public health administrators an opportunity to evaluate their perceptions of African Americans' health and social needs as depicted in documented public health data with the perceptions from the African American community and the type of public health initiative that will truly work in the African American community.

The African American Health Researcher

Here are five cultural health empowerment strategies for the African American health researcher:

1. In the conceptualization of a research project that is designed to conduct research among African Americans, use a model (medical anthropology and/or public health) that allows for the investigation of cultural issues equally with the health and social issues of your project.

2. Once the general research plan is completed, brainstorm your approach with other African American and non-African American researchers who share a common approach to health care research.
3. Develop a diverse team of experienced and newly trained African American professionals along with African American community activists and key African American informants who will work closely in developing a comprehensive research project.
4. Collect preliminary data from a variety of documented cultural, social, and medical sources. Using the applied medical anthropological strategies for conducting research, interview key community leaders and community residents who will offer key cultural health information to your project.
5. Share the results of each phase of your study with all those who are involved—particularly the African American community.

The primary purpose of this cultural health empowerment strategy is to encourage the African American health researcher to use a model that is more culturally appropriate for the African American population and to develop a team of primarily African American health researchers, non-African American health researchers, and key African American community leaders who can work together to conduct a comprehensive, quality, and ethical research study.

The Non-African American Health Researcher

Here are five cultural health empowerment strategies for the non-African American health researcher who has had little or limited exposure to the African American community.

1. Conduct basic background cultural, historical, and contemporary research on the culture of African Americans nationally and locally. Try not to generalize about the African American community either nationally or locally with regards to health, social, economic, and cultural issues. Consider taking a cultural sensitivity course/seminar.
2. In the conceptualization of a research project that is designed to conduct research among African Americans, use a model (medical anthropology and/or public health) that allows for the investigation of cultural issues equally with the health and social issues of your project.
3. Once the general research plan is completed, brainstorm and include several African American health researchers who share a common approach to health care research. Allow others to assist with the design and implementation of the project.
4. Develop a diverse team of experienced and newly trained African American and non-African American professionals along with African American community activists and key African American informants who will work closely in developing a comprehensive research project. Assure the research

team about the ethical guidelines of the project and attempt to solve any uncertainty.
5. Using the applied medical anthropological strategies for conducting re-
    search, interview key community leaders and community residents who will
    offer key cultural health information for your project. Share the results of
    each phase of your study with all those who are involved—particularly the
    African American community.

The primary purpose of this cultural health empowerment strategy is to encourage the non-African American health researcher to learn about the diversity of
African American culture and to conduct an ethical, quality, comprehensive, and
culturally relativistic research project.

CONCLUSION

Culture and its relationship to health are the focus of this book. As stated in
Chapter 1 and throughout this text, medical anthropology views health from a
biopsychosociocultural perspective. Biology, psychology, sociology, and culture
are all combined in this holistic approach for the purpose of diagnosing and
treating an individual from a comprehensive perspective.

In fact, I suggest that all of us should reorient our approach to the biopsychosociocultural model. That is, culture, not biological, psychological, or so-
ciological factors, should be the focal point to this model. Interestingly, if more
health care researchers and health care professionals viewed *culture* differently
and recognized its direct relationship to health care, then more health care
problems would be resolved and prevented.

With regard to African American health, the biopsychosociocultural perspective is appropriate for many African Americans due to the fact that it fits
their perception of health and illness. Health and illness has always been viewed
from a holistic perspective for many African Americans in the past and the present. Moreover, culture has always played a significant role in this view of health
and illness.

Thus, *culture*, as it has in the past and the present, will be the driving force or
the key factor in solving many of the health problems that all of us will face in
the future!

POST-EVALUATION QUESTIONS

1. Why do you need specific cultural health strategies for different cultural
    groupings within the African American population?

2. What can health care professionals, health researchers, and public health
    administrators learn from developing specific strategies for the African
    American population?

3.   Why are cultural health empowerment strategies needed for African
        Americans today and in the future?

REFERENCES

Adams, P., C. Scholenborn, A. Moss, NCHS, C. Warren, and L Kann. 1995.
        Health-Risk Behaviors Among Our Nation's Youth: United States,
        1992. Washington, DC: U.S. Department of Health and Human Serv-
        ices.
American Cancer Society. 1998. *Cancer Facts & Figures–1998.* Atlanta, GA:
        American Cancer Society.
Bailey, Eric. "Hypertension: An Ethnomedical Analysis of Detroit African
        American Treatment Patterns." *Human Organization* 50: 287–296.
Blendon, R., L. Aiken, H. Freeman, and C. Correy. 1989. "Access to Medical
        Care for Black and White Americans. A Matter of Continuing Con-
        cern." *Journal of the American Medical Association* 261: 278–281.
Braithwaite, Ronald, Bianchi, Cynthia and Sandra Taylor. 1994. "Ethnographic
        Approach to Community Organization and Health Empowerment."
        Health Education Quarterly 21: 407–416.
Braithwaite, Ronald and Ngina Lythcott. 1989. "Community Empowerment as a
        Strategy for Health Promotion for Black and Other Minority Popula-
        tions." *Journal of the American Medical Association* 261: 282–283.
Brangman, Sharon. 1995. "African American Elders: Implications for Health
        Care Providers." *Clinics in Geriatric Medicine* 11: 15–23.
Brawley, Otis. 1998. "Prostate Cancer and Black Men." *Seminars in Urologic*
        Oncology 16: 184–186.
Brawley, Otis and Nayda Figueroa-Valles. 1998. "Prostate Cancer Research and
        the National Cancer Institute." *Seminars in Urologic Oncology* 16:
        235–240.
Collins, M. 1997. "Increasing Prostate Cancer Awareness in African American
        Men." *Oncology Nursing Forum* Jan/Feb 24: 91–95.
Curry, R., J. Moen, S. Morris, and L. Scheivelhud. 1994. "Community-Directed
        Cancer Screening Program." *Cancer Practice* 2: 256–263.
Demark-Wahnefried, W., J. McClelland, M. Campbell, K. Hoben, J. Lashley, C.
        Graves, B. Motsinger, and B. Rimer. 1998. "Awareness of Cancer-
        Related Programs and Services among Rural African Americans."
        Journal of the National Medical Association 90: 197–202.
Erwin, Deborah, Thea Spatz, and Carolyn Turturro. 1992. "Development of an
        African American Role Model Intervention to Increase Breast Self-
        Examination and Mammography." *Journal of Cancer Education* 7:
        311–319.
Forte, Deirdra. 1995. "Community-Based Breast Cancer Intervention Program
        for Older African American Women in Beauty Salons." *Public Health*
        Reports 110: 179–183.

Freedman, Tovia. 1998. "Why Don't They Come to Pike Street and Ask Us?" Black American Women's Health Concerns." *Social Science and Medicine* 47: 941–947.

Geiger, H. 1972. "A Health Center in Mississippi: A Case Study in Social Medicine." In *Medicine in a Changing Society*. L. Corey, S. Saltman and M. Epstein, eds. St. Louis: C.V. Mosby.

Guidry, J. et al. 1998. "Cultural Sensitivity and Readability of Breast and Prostate Printed Cancer Education Materials Targeting African Americans." *Journal of the National Medical Association* 90: 165–169.

Harris, Y. et al. 1996. "Why African Americans May Not Be Participating in Clinical Trials." *Journal of National Medical Association* 88: 630–634.

Hazuda, Helen. 1997. "Minority Issues in Alzheimer Disease Outcomes Research." *Alzheimer Disease and Associated Disorders* 11: 156–161.

Jennings, Kathleen. 1996. "Getting Black Women to Screen for Cancer: Incorporating Health Beliefs Into Practice." *Journal of the American Academy of Nursing Practitioners* 8: 53–59.

Johnson, Ernest et al. 1996. "Obesity and Hypertension Among African Americans: Do African American Primary Care Providers Address These Conditions When Secondary to Primary Illness?" *Journal of the National Medical Association* 88: 225–229.

Kumanyika, S. 1990. "Diet and Chronic Disease Issues for Minority Populations." *Journal of Nutrition Education* 22: 89–96.

———. 1994. "Obesity in Minority Populations: An Epidemiologic Assessment." *Obesity Research* 2: 166–182.

Levinson, S. et al. 1985. "Ethnic Differences in Blood Pressure and Heart Rate of Chicago School Children." *American Journal of Epidemiology* 122: 366–377.

Mandelblatt, J., M. Traxler, P. Lakin, and P. Kanetsky. 1993. "Breast and Cervical Cancer Screening of Poor, Elderly Black Women: Clinical Results and Implications." *American Journal of Preventive Medicine* 9: 133–137.

Martin, Judy and Carol Panicucci. 1996. "Health-Related Practices and Priorities: The Health Behaviors and Beliefs of Community-Living Black Older Women." *Journal of Gerontological Nursing* 22: 41–48.

Meyers, R. et al. 1994. "Receptivity of African American Men to Prostate Cancer Screening." *Urology* 43: 480–487.

Michielutte, R., M. Dignan, H. Wells, L. Young, D. Jackson, and P. Sharp. 1989. "Development of a Community Cancer Education Program: The Forsyth County, NC Cervical Cancer Prevention Project." *Public Health Report* 104: 542–551.

Mouton, Charles, Johnson, Mark and David Cole. 1995. "Ethical Considerations with African American Elders." *Ethnogeriatrics* 11: 113–129.

Mouton, Charles, S. Harris, S. Rovi, P. Solorzano, and M. Johnson. 1997. "Barriers to Black Women's Participation in Cancer Clinical Trials." *Journal of the National Medical Association* 89: 721–727.

National Center for Health Statistics. 1995. *Health-Risk Behaviors Among Our Nation's Youth: United States, 1992*: Atlanta, GA: The Centers for Disease Control and Prevention.

Otten, W. et al. 1990. "The Effect of Known Risk Factors on the Excess Mortality of Black Adults in the United States." *Journal of American Medical Association* 263: 845–850.

Pachter, Lee. 1994. "Culture and Clinical Care: Folk Illness Beliefs and Behaviors and Their Implications for Health Care Delivery." *Journal of American Medical Association* 271: 690-694.

Pinn, Vivian. 1995. "Status of Women's Health Research: Where Are African American Women?" *Journal of National Black Nurses Association* 8–19.

Post, Douglas and Wilburn Weddington. 1997. "The Impact of Culture on Physician Stress and Coping." *Journal of the National Medical Association* 89: 585–590.

Powell I., L. Heilbrun, P. Littrup, A. Franklin, J. Parzuchowski, D. Gelfand, and W. Sakr. 1997. "Outcome of African American Men Screened for Prostate Cancer; The Detroit Education and Early Detection Study." *Journal of Urology* 158: 146–149.

Price, James et al. 1993. "Prostate Cancer: Perceptions of African American Males." *Journal of the National Medical Association* 85: 941–947.

Rosenberg, Lynn, Adams-Campbell, Lucille and Julie Palmer. 1995. "The Black Women's Health Study: A Follow-up Study for Causes and Preventions of Illness." *Journal of American Medical Women's Association* 50: 56–58.

Russell, Kathleen and Nancy Jewell. 1992. "Cultural Impact of Health-Care Access: Challenges for Improving the Health of African Americans." *Journal of Community Health Nursing* 9: 161–169.

Stolley, Melinda and Marian Fitzgibbon. 1997. "Effects of an Obesity Prevention Program on the Eating Behavior of African American Mothers and Daughters." *Health Education and Behavior* 24: 152–164.

Suarez, L., D. Nichols, L. Pulley, C. Brady, and A. McAlister. 1993. "Local Health Departments Implement a Theory-Based Model to Increase Breast and Cervical Cancer Screening." *Journal of Cancer Education* 108: 477–482.

Suarez, L., L. Lloyd, N. Weiss, T. Rainbolt, and L. Pulley. 1994. "Effect of Social Networks on Cancer-Screening Behavior of Older Mexican-American Women." *Journal of the National Cancer Institute* 86: 775–779.

Tatum, Cathy, A. Wilson, M. Dignan, E. Paskett, and R. Velez. 1997. "Development and Implementation of Outreach Strategies for Breast and Cervical Cancer Prevention among African American Women." *Journal of Cancer Prevention* 12: 43–50.

Toliver-Weddington, Gloria. 1990. "Cultural Considerations in the Treatment of Craniofacial Malformations in African Americans." *Cleft Palate Journal* 27: 289-293.

U.S. Department of Health & Human Services. 1997. *Health United States 1996-97.* Washington, DC: National Center for Health Statistics. DHHS Publication No. 97–1232.

———. 1998. *Healthy People 2010.* Office of Disease Prevention & Health Promotion. Washington D.C.: U.S. Government Printing Office.

Voorhees, Carolyn et al. 1996. "Heart, Body, and Soul: Impact of Church-Based Smoking Cessation Interventions on Readiness to Quit." *Preventive Medicine* 25: 277–285.

Walcott-McQuigg, Jacqueline et al. 1995. "Psychosocial Factors Influencing Weight Control Behavior of African American Women." *Western Journal of Nursing Research* 17: 502–520.

Weinrich, Sally, D. Holdford, M. Boyd, D. Creanga, A. Johnson, M. Frank-Stromborg, and M. Weinrich. 1998. "Prostate Cancer Education in African American Churches." *Public Health Nursing* 15: 188–195.

Whitehead, Tony. 1997. "Urban Low-Income African American Men, HIV/AIDS, and Gender Identity." *Medical Anthropology Quarterly* 11: 411–447.

Witness Project. 1998. *The Witness Project Manual.* Little Rock, AR: The Centers for Disease Control and Prevention.

Yancy, A. and L. Walden. 1994. "Stimulating Cancer Screening among Latinas and African American Women: A Community Case Study." *Journal of Cancer Education* 9: 46–52.

WEB SITES OF SIGNIFICANCE

Healthy People 2000

http://odphp.osophs.dhhs.gov/pubs/hp2000/

Healthy People 2000: Progress Report for Black Americans

http://odphp.osophs.dhhs.gov/pubs/hp2000/pdf/prog_rvw/prgblack.pdf

Healthy People 2010

http://web.health.gov/healthypeople

Index

About the Author

ERIC J. BAILEY is a medical anthropologist with the U.S. Department of Health and Human Services.

ISBN 0-89789-592-4

90000>

EAN

9 780897 895927

HARDCOVER BAR CODE